COLLEAGUES IN DISCOVERY

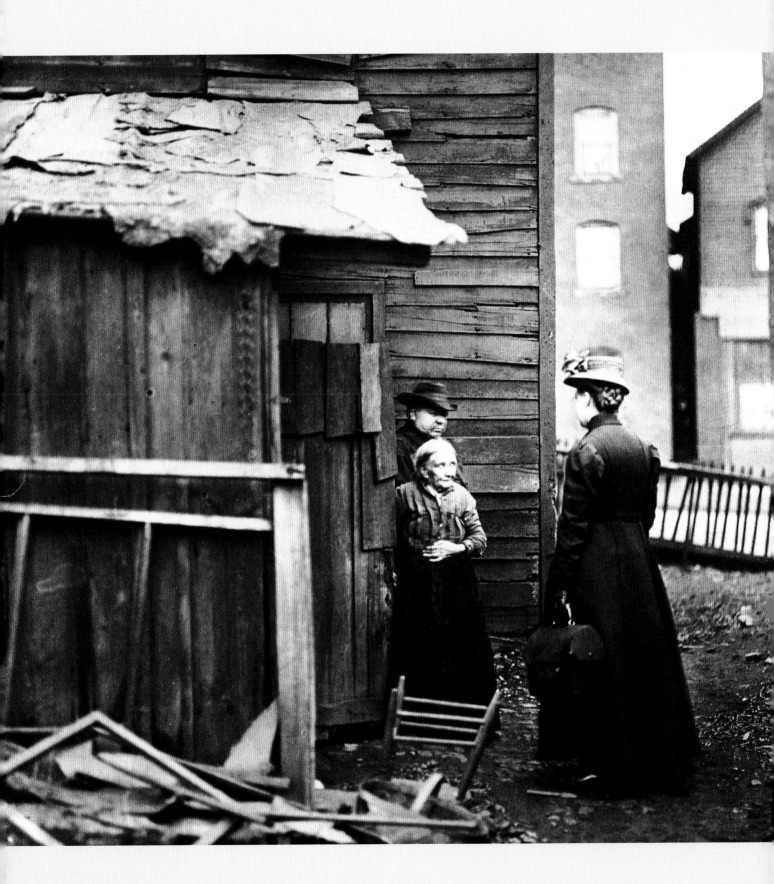

An American Thoracic Society Perspective

National Jewish Health
Medical Library

COLLEAGUES IN DISCOVERY
One Hundred Years of Improving Respiratory Health

by Joseph Wallace

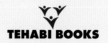
TEHABI BOOKS

Unrestricted grant provided by these Patron sponsors:
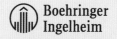 Boehringer Ingelheim
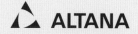 ALTANA

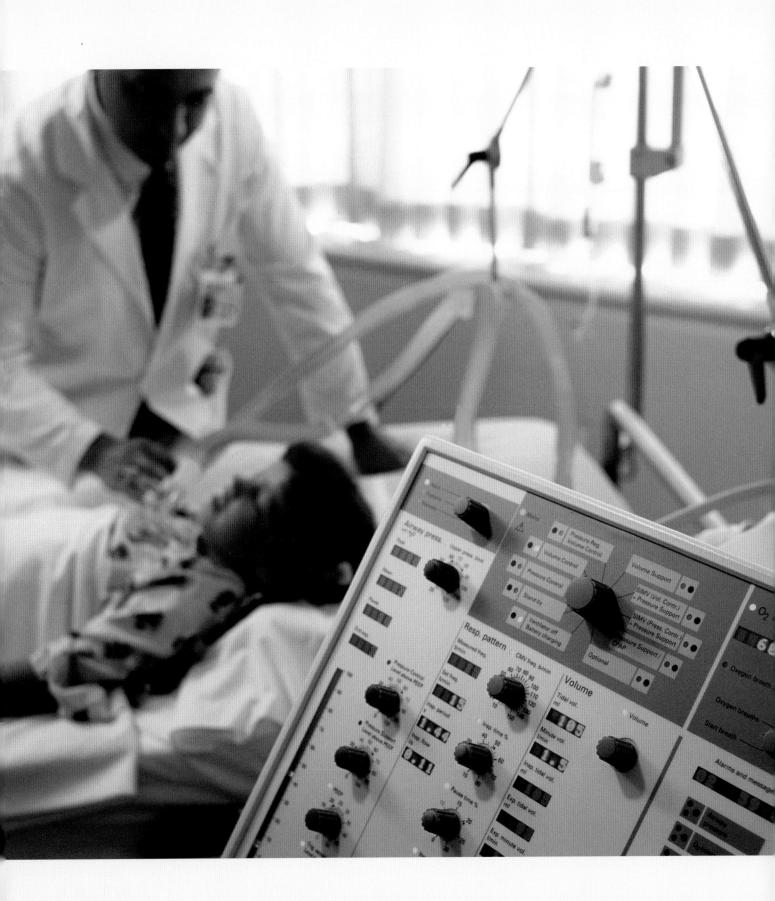

TABLE OF CONTENTS

Previous page: A nurse visits a family living in an urban tenement early in the twentieth century. It was a time when tuberculosis swept through such crowded, airless tenements—but nurses and doctors alike had little to offer those who were ill.

Opposite: A young patient is hooked up to a respirator, one of the many innovations that has wrought a revolution in respiratory medicine.

ACKNOWLEDGMENTS

In 1905 a group of physicians founded an organization to share experiences caring for patients in tuberculosis sanatoriums. Named the American Sanatorium Association, it has grown and evolved over the past one 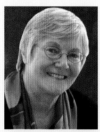 hundred years to become the American Thoracic Society. Accordingly, in 2005, we celebrate our centennial, "100 Years of *A*dvances in *T*reatment and *S*cience of Respiratory Diseases."

Since 1905 there has been remarkable progress in the identification, treatment, and prevention of lung and lung-related diseases. Disciplines that could not have been imagined in 1905 are mainstream for the American 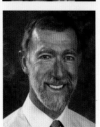 Thoracic Society in 2005—for example, exciting new domains such as the genetics, genomics, and proteomics of respiratory diseases are now a growing and critical part of the fight against lung disease. The name, mission, and composition of the American Thoracic Society have changed over the past hundred years to reflect this evolution.

The idea for this book came from a group of American Thoracic Society members who planned for the Centennial. This "Birthday Bash Committee" included Sonia Buist, M.D., Randy Curtis, M.D., Colleen Richardson, Sharon Rounds, M.D., Dean Schraufnagel, M.D., Martin Tobin, M.D., Gerry Turino, M.D., Peter Wagner, M.D., and John Walsh, along with several ATS staff members—Carl Booberg, Cathy Carlomagno, Gary Ewart, Rebecca Fournier, and Graham Nelan. We were fortunate to engage Tehabi Books, well known for producing beautiful books, and Joe Wallace, an accomplished author.

Colleagues in Discovery: One Hundred Years of Improving Respiratory Health celebrates a century of progress in respiratory research and its application to clinical medicine. It is not a history of the American Thoracic

Society per se. Rather, our goal has been to provide an overview of major advances over the past century and the role of Society members in this progress. We realize that it is not possible to list in one volume all the achievements and events and people of the past hundred years. Accordingly, we understand that some readers will likely be able to identify developments that could not be included.

A project of this magnitude requires the input of many people. We wish to acknowledge the contributions of the many Society members who provided important information and images for the book. In addition, we thank the American Lung Association for use of materials from their archives.

Finally, we gratefully acknowledge the financial support of our corporate sponsors who provided unrestricted grants to the American Thoracic Society for development, production, and distribution of this book. These sponsors include Altana Pharma, Boehringer-Ingelheim Pharmaceuticals, Inc., Genentech, Inc./Novartis Pharmaceuticals Corporation, and Merck & Co., Inc.

The American Thoracic Society is proud to have played an important role in the remarkable advances in respiratory science and medicine over the last one hundred years and stands ready to serve patients, healthcare professionals, scientists, and policymakers through the coming century. It is clear that much remains to be learned and accomplished in the ongoing battle against respiratory diseases. We hope that this book will serve as an inspiration to join that battle for all who read it.

SHARON ROUNDS
PRESIDENT
AMERICAN THORACIC SOCIETY
2004–2005

PETER WAGNER
PRESIDENT
AMERICAN THORACIC SOCIETY
2005–2006

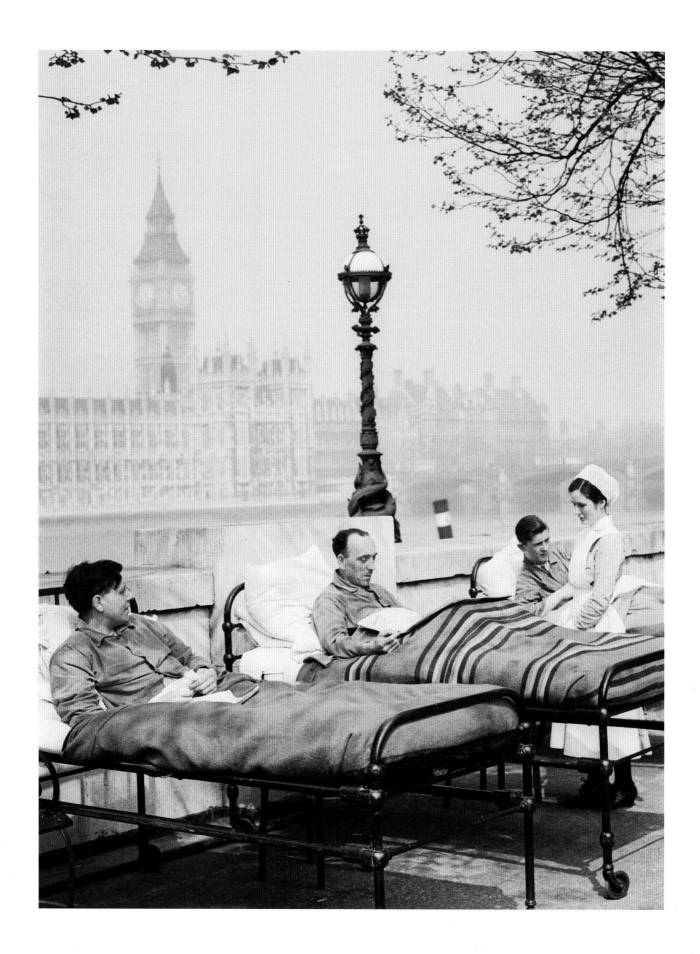

CHAPTER ONE

A Consuming Concern

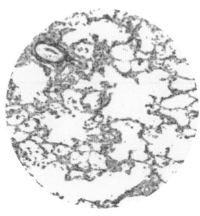

The normal human lung. X-rays and more advanced scanning techniques have made it far easier to detect infection with *Mycobacteria tuberculosis* and other microbes far earlier than was possible a century ago.

"Any important disease whose causality is murky, and for which treatment is ineffectual, tends to be awash in significance."

—SUSAN SONTAG, AUTHOR (1933–PRESENT)

DESPERATE TIMES, THE OFT-USED SAYING GOES, call for desperate measures.

For the practice of medicine in the nineteenth and twentieth centuries, no truer words have ever been spoken. If ever there was a desperate time in the history of human health, a time calling for unparalleled bravery, creativity, and academic and medical brilliance, it was those crucial two hundred years.

The impetus for this turning point in history was a single epidemic disease: tuberculosis. It was a disease so rampant, so widely feared, that it helped spur a revolution in medical practice. Old habits were abandoned, old philosophies were revised, old tenets were discarded—not only in the struggle to understand and treat tuberculosis, but in medicine as a whole.

But before physicians could figure out how to confront an age-old disease that seemed capable of bringing civilization to its knees, they had to gain a far deeper understanding of the structure and function of the lungs than had been achieved in the previous two millennia.

The Body's Bellows: Early Knowledge of the Lung

From at least the time of the great Greek physician Hippocrates (460–377 B.C.), medical practitioners have understood that the lungs play a crucial role in the successful functioning of the human body. The question for them was: What exactly did the lungs *do*? Even as Hippocrates became the first to employ (or at least to write about) tube thoracostomy, the insertion of a tube into the pleural sac to drain pus

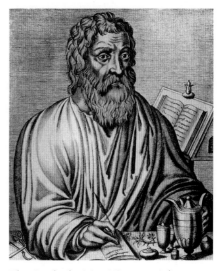

The Greek physician Hippocrates, known as "the father of medicine." Believing that the body's four humours (blood, phlegm, and yellow and black bile) were the primary seats of disease, he understood little of the structure or function of the lung—or of the diseases that affected it.

Opposite: Prior to the first effective antimicrobial medicines in the 1940s, treatment for tuberculosis patients relied on rest and fresh air, as shown in this 1936 photograph taken at St. Thomas' Hospital opposite the Houses of Parliament in London.

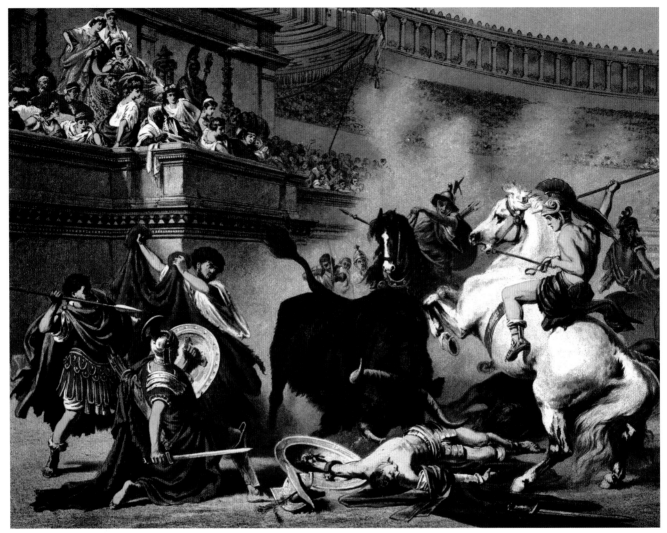

and relieve a patient's discomfort, he and other early practitioners understood little of the purpose of the lungs.

Nearly five hundred years after Hippocrates, the great Greek physician-philosopher Galen looked deeper into the physiology of the lung. Born in A.D. 130, Galen was a child of privilege who as a teenager became a *therapeutes*, or attendant, to the healing god Asclepius. The story has it that the god himself visited Galen's father in a dream and instructed him to make the boy a physician.

As a strict follower of Hippocrates's writings, Galen believed that the main purpose of respiration was humoral heating and cooling—that the lungs, in effect, were organic bellows designed to stoke and control the temperature of the blood. "Blood passing through the lungs absorbed from the inhaled air, the quality of heat, which it then carried into the left heart," he wrote, adding that the lungs also cooled over-heated blood via "the substance of the air."

The idea that air in the lungs served mainly as a cooling device remained paramount for centuries. In the late fifteenth century,

The dreadful injuries that struck gladiators in combat in ancient Rome provided a rare opportunity for the Greek physician-philosopher Galen (130–200 A.D.), who for several years served as physician to the gladiators. His explorations of the lung led him to believe that blood, passing through the lungs, maintained the body's optimum heat by either absorbing heat from or releasing it to the outside air.

Leonardo da Vinci modified this belief to add cleansing as well. He studied lung physiology carefully, and learned that the substance of the lung "is spongy and if you press it, it yields to the force which compresses it, and if the force is removed, it increases again to its original size." The purpose of this elasticity, he believed, was to cleanse the body: "From the heart, impurities or 'sooty vapors' are carried back to the lung by way of the pulmonary artery, to be exhaled into the outer air."

Yet even scientists as brilliant as Hippocrates and da Vinci, while understanding that ancient theories did not explain everything, struggled to come up with a satisfying explanation of exactly what it was that the lungs did by drawing air into the body. It took the sixteenth-century German philosopher, mystic, and medical reformer Paracelsus to look at the lungs from a different angle—and in doing so, to peel off the blinders that had hindered investigators for more than a thousand years.

Ingeniously, Paracelsus focused on diseases of the lungs. Though this seems like an elementary concept now, it was revolutionary at the time. In his research on mine workers, Paracelsus identified a link between the lungs and the outside world that no one had ever considered before. As the disease now known as silicosis showed, the lungs were capable of doing more than just drawing in air to cool the heart. They were capable of drawing in substances that caused disease as well.

By the seventeenth century, the great British physician William Harvey had incorporated and developed all previous findings about lung physiology. His work detailing the body's unified circulatory system and the pulmonary role in that system remains a marvel of intelligence and academic rigor.

In his *Lectures on the Whole of Anatomy* (1653), Harvey asserted the primacy of the lungs over the liver—and even over the heart. "[Nothing] is especially so necessary, neither sensation nor ailment," he wrote. "Life and respiration are complementary. There is nothing living which does not breathe nor anything breathing which does not live."

The work of Hippocrates, da Vinci, Paracelsus, and Harvey slowly but steadily advanced our understanding of the lungs, their function, and the diseases that afflict them. Yet more than two thousand years of effort seemed but a prelude when, in the eighteenth century, physicians had to confront tuberculosis, the disease that proved William Harvey's bold statement of more than a century earlier: "Life and respiration are complementary." When tuberculosis took away respiration, life came to a painful and premature end.

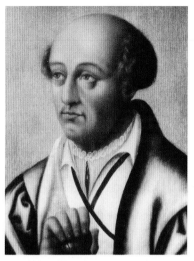

The Swiss-born German physician and alchemist Paracelsus (1493–1541) was one of the first to reject the centuries-old humoral theory of medicine—a break from the past that allowed him to identify silicosis and congenital syphilis, among other diseases. Paracelsus's belief that specific diseases called for specific remedies laid the groundwork for modern medicine.

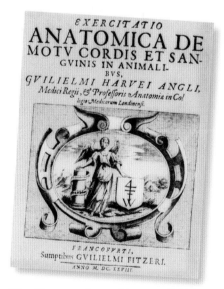

The title page of one of the great British physician William Harvey's treatises. The brilliant Harvey (1578–1657) revolutionized prevailing scientific views of the lungs and their central role in sustaining life.

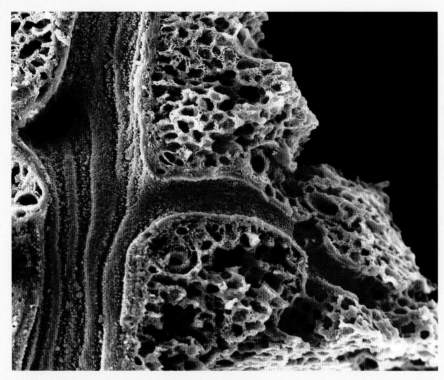

A microscopic image of the airways and alveoli of the lung. A miracle of engineering, the lungs act in concert with the diaphragm and chest-wall muscles, the circulatory system, and the brain, to permit the rapid and efficient gas exchange that allows life to exist.

How the Lung Works

The main function of the lungs is to bring the body's blood into as close contact as possible with the air—and, in doing so, to allow rapid and efficient gas exchange. During gas exchange, carbon dioxide, produced as a waste product by the body, is given up into the atmosphere, while fresh oxygen is absorbed by the blood.

Gas exchange is achieved by a complex interaction of the lungs with the central nervous system, the diaphragm and chest-wall muscles, and the circulatory system. It occurs in the alveoli, where air is separated from the blood by as few as two cells. The importance and extent of gas exchange is shown by the fact that the adult body contains about 300 million alveoli. The surface area covered by these alveoli within the lungs can measure eighty square meters, about the size of a tennis court. The body's entire blood volume passes through the lungs each minute, even when the body is in a resting state.

Air—as much as ten thousand liters per day—first enters the body through the trachea, or windpipe. It is carried down to smaller tubes called bronchi, and then into even smaller ones called bronchioles, which are controlled by muscles so that their diameter can be varied. The air, finally reaching the alveoli, has been warmed by the body and filtered of particles and other impurities by tiny hairs in the bronchi and bronchioles. In addition, specialized cells within the lungs, called alveolar macrophages ingest particulate matter and bacteria and thereby cleanse the lung.

While the conducting airways (trachea, bronchi, bronchioles) and gas-exchange portions (alveoli) are the central facets of lung structure, a variety of other cells also participate in lung function. Goblet cells and bronchial submucosal glands, for example, produce mucous essential to loosening material carried into the lungs during breathing; Clara cells produce a watery secretion that helps both with clearance and reduction of surface tension in small airways; and ciliated columnar cells use their cilia to remove the accumulated material from the lungs.

Other cells, including Kulchitzky cells, are fascinatingly complex in structure, yet continue to present challenges to investigators seeking to determine their exact purpose. Despite extraordinary advances in our understanding of lung structure and function, clearly much remains to be learned.

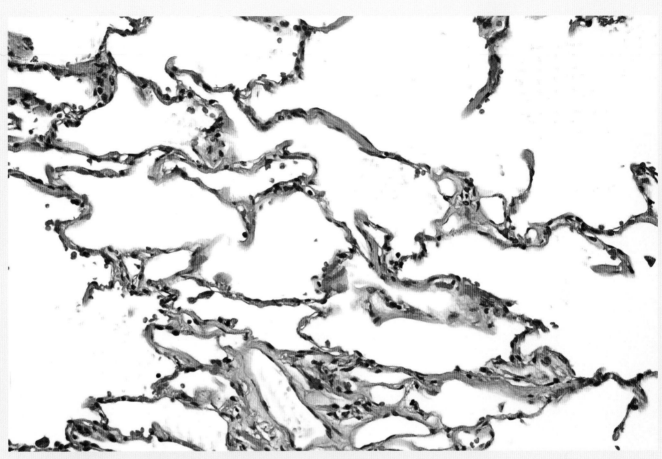

Some of the many alveoli of a healthy lung. As many as ten thousand liters of air travel through ever-smaller passages until reaching the alveoli, where it comes in contact with the bloodstream, permitting the exchange of oxygen and carbon dioxide.

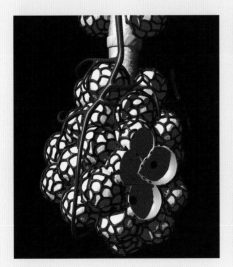

This model of the acinus of a lung shows a bronchiole (center), along with alveoli and other structures.

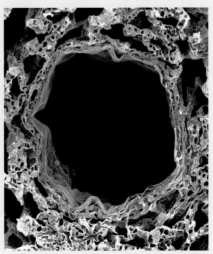

A closer look at a bronchiole, a conducting airway that also filters the air before it reaches the alveoli.

Tuberculosis: A Scourge of History

It is likely that the first hominid walked the earth no more than about five million years ago. How much earlier did the first tuberculosis bacillus appear? Millions of years, certainly, probably tens of millions, and possibly hundreds of millions of years earlier, far before the first mammals evolved. Its home turf was most likely the soil or underwater mud, where it was inhaled or ingested by animals while feeding.

It is also likely that some form of tuberculosis affected early hominids, just as other strains affected other species, although no such evidence has yet been found among the fossil record of early man. We do know for sure that, in the earliest days of recorded history, the disease had already dug an important foothold in societies around the world. Tuberculosis is a disease that can affect many areas of the body, but its most common and distinctive form is a pulmonary disease that has also been termed *consumption* or *phthisis*. All types of tuberculosis, however, are usually spread through respiratory means, and all areas of the world have been infected.

Skeletons dating back six thousand years that have been uncovered in Europe show signs of tuberculosis. Egyptian mummies and tomb paintings dating back to the same era also reveal the telltale skeletal signs of active tuberculosis, including the "hunchback" and other skeletal changes. As A. J. E. Cave reported in the *British Journal of Tuberculosis* in 1939, one mummified priest's body even showed the track of pus that had leaked from a tubercular spinal abscess.

Other ancient cultures recognized the disease later known as tuberculosis. The disease was well known among the Hindus of India, and is mentioned and described in the holy Hindu Vetas, which date back nearly four thousand years. Under the name *shachepheth* (from a word meaning "to waste away"), it is mentioned twice in the Old Testament.

The pre-Columbian New World was by no means free of the disease. Unlike smallpox, measles, and other diseases, tuberculosis did not arrive with European explorers. Skeletal remains reveal that far before Columbus arrived, the disease was already endemic—and sometimes epidemic—among the Indians of northern North America, the Maya in Central America, and the Andean people of Peru.

A disease so widespread and dramatic in its symptoms couldn't help but catch the attention of physicians, mystics, and philosophers in cultures worldwide. For more than a thousand years, they came up with attempts at treatment—some logical, some hopeless, but none able to contend with a disease that seemed impregnable.

As early as the eleventh century, the Islamic physician Avicenna was recommending dry air and fresh milk as a treatment for the disease. Other

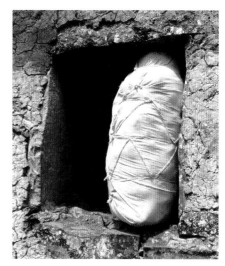

A thousand-year-old mummy unearthed in Peru. Examination of such mummies reveals that tuberculosis has likely been present in both the Old and New Worlds for millennia. The disease may, in fact, have predated the arrival of *Homo sapiens* on earth.

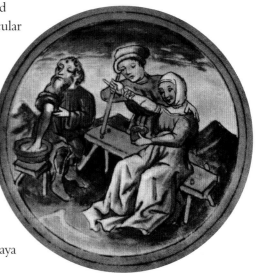

Bad blood, circa 1350. Helpless to defeat the "white plague" of tuberculosis, medieval physicians resorted to treatments such as a quiver that was bare of arrows. Here, a physician bleeds a patient.

Arab physicians sought to relieve the symptoms of tuberculosis with camphor and sugar distilled from grapes. A plethora of other cures were attempted—from tinctures of gold to bleeding to the healing touch of kings (which was only fair, since scrofula, a form of tuberculosis characterized by draining infected lymph nodes in the neck was known as "The King's Evil")—but the disease still took a dreadful toll.

In the mid-seventeenth century, consumption was responsible for 20 percent of all recorded deaths in London, was tearing through cities on the Continent, and was an increasing presence in North America as well. But as an epidemic, it was just getting started. By the end of the eighteenth century, the disease's long-honed survival skills, society's lack of knowledge about its cause and effective treatments, and cramped, industrial conditions came together to create a health disaster that is almost beyond imagination.

The White Plague

Just how catastrophic was the tuberculosis epidemic from the turn of the nineteenth century through the middle of the twentieth? No one knows for sure how many people died of the disease worldwide during those years, but Frank Ryan's estimate in his book *The Forgotten Plague* seems reasonable: around one billion. One billion men, women, and children fell victim to a microscopic bacillus that had an affinity for traveling through the air, was carried on currents of wind or a cough or sneeze, and then lodged itself in the lungs before multiplying. A billion individuals who lived under conditions conducive to the spread of disease by respiratory means.

Until a few hundred years ago, most humans had always lived in small towns or the country. What cities existed were small, and even if a disease outbreak occurred, it was unlikely to spread from village to village, given how few people traveled any great distance. So while tuberculosis had been widespread and well known for centuries, conditions had usually prevented it from reaching epidemic ferocity. It was a steady killer, but rarely as virulent as shorter-lived epidemics like those caused by the bubonic plague or smallpox.

But then conditions changed. At the turn of the nineteenth century, population growth, the Industrial Revolution, famine in rural areas, and other factors led people to congregate in European and American cities. London, Paris, New York, and other metropolises grew exponentially in size; New York City's population, for example, grew from less than five thousand in 1700 to two hundred and fifty thousand by 1820.

Great numbers of city dwellers lived in dark, crowded tenements, and worked packed together in unventilated industrial factories (dubbed "dark satanic mills" by the poet William Blake). While it was almost

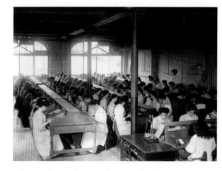

The Industrial Revolution that began at the turn of the nineteenth century allowed tuberculosis and other respiratory diseases to spread rapidly. Vulnerable workers were packed into airless workspaces (like this cigarette-rolling factory) in which pathogens thrived. The result was a tuberculosis epidemic that shook the foundations of society in Europe and the United States alike.

Following spread: With the rise of crowded cities (including Paris, pictured here) in the nineteenth century, tuberculosis found conditions ripe for explosive spread.

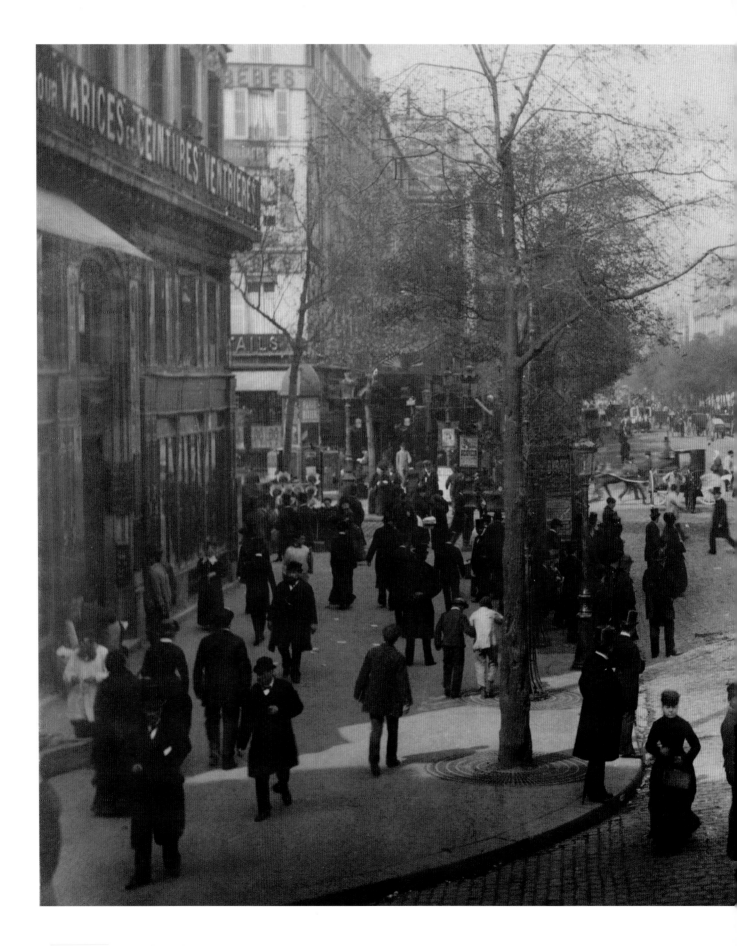

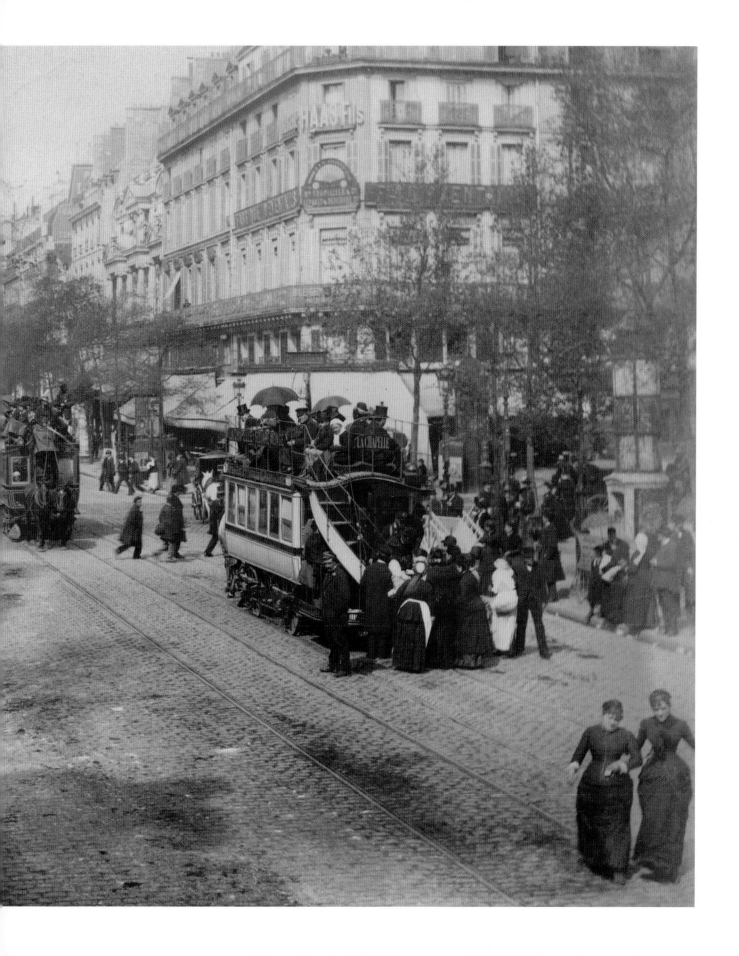

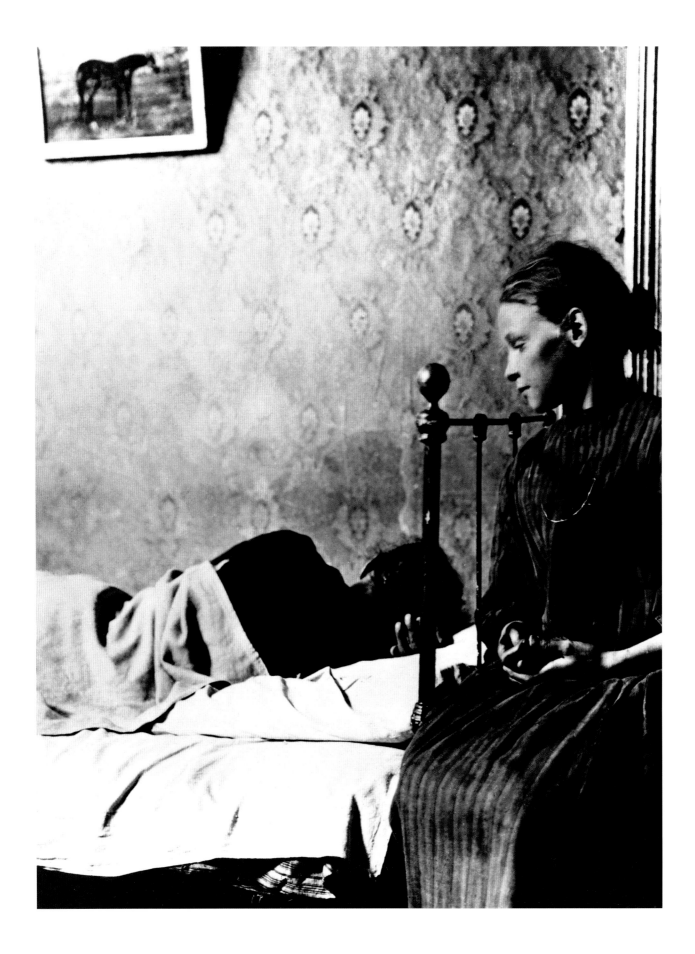

impossible to find open space, fresh air, or clean water, it was easy to rub shoulders—and share air—with someone who was infected with tuberculosis.

By the beginning of the nineteenth century, the death rate from tuberculosis was about seven million people a year worldwide. Fifty million had open infection, and at least 500 million (half the world's population) had been exposed to the disease. London, New York, and other cities were burying hundreds of victims each day, and yet the epidemic was still dawning.

Vulnerable tenement-dwellers were far from the only targets of the disease's spread. Tuberculosis was no respecter of class, wealth, or breeding. It was, after all, called "The King's Evil," and well into the twentieth century, one after another brilliant or beloved cultural icon perished from the white plague, along with more than a fair share of royalty.

The roll call of the famous people who died from what John Bunyan called "the captain of all these men of death" remains shocking. Robert Louis Stevenson. Anton Chekhov. Honoré Balzac. Emily, Anne, and Charlotte Brontë. Frédéric Chopin. Edgar Allan Poe. George Orwell. D. H. Lawrence. John Keats. Louis XVII of France. No one was safe from a disease whose cause remained a mystery, and whose treatments seemed to do no good whatsoever.

A Profession at a Loss

The medical profession was ill-equipped to confront the epidemic. As Katherine Ott put it in her book *Fevered Lives*, medical practice until the late 1800s was "virtually a free-for-all. No one approach predominated: a consumptive might consult a homeopath, allopath, hydropath, osteopath, or a practitioner of any of dozens of other more obscure medical theories, including an aging but impenitent phrenologist. The anarchy in medicine allowed for all manner of theory and practice, and experts on consumption were drawn from the ranks of ministers, moralists, physicians, and astute neighbors."

But it almost didn't matter which modality a patient chose: they were all useless in the face of tuberculosis. Chopin, writing to a friend from the island of Mallorca, said, "I have been sick as a dog the last two weeks; I caught cold in spite of 18 degrees [Celsius] of heat, roses, oranges, palms, figs and the three most famous doctors on the island. One sniffed at what I spat up, the second tapped where I spat it from, the third poked about and listened how I spat it. One said I had died, the second that I am dying, and the third that I shall die."

This was a typical medical response. Like Chopin, other patients took what they could get. They accepted the same treatments that had "worked" for their parents, depending on prayer or magic or bleeding by leeches to recover from tuberculosis, and other diseases ranging from syphilis

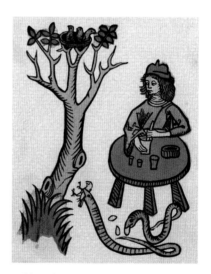

A fifteenth-century apothecary gathered his potions from wherever he could find them— including, in this case, the flesh of snakes that had eaten birds and eggs.

Opposite: The tuberculosis epidemic was no respecter of race, age, or class and often took parents from their children before their time.

to cancer. In Europe in the mid-1800s, the average life expectancy was less than forty years.

Making matters even worse were the hydra-like characteristics of tuberculosis patients: crumbling spines, grotesque thickening and reddening of the skin on the face *(lupus vulgaris)*, convulsions in the young. Tuberculosis's pulmonary form, consumption, had a multitude of symptoms as well: weight loss, fever, coughing and expectoration, including the coughing up of blood and fragments of lung tubercles. In fact, the condition called *tuberculosis* in the nineteenth century referred specifically to this last symptom, not to the disease as a whole, but eventually became a way to describe a disease that had many names over time.

It's no surprise that there were people at the time who believed the white plague was destined to keep spreading, claiming more and more lives until civilization itself came to an end. As entire neighborhoods were stricken and entire families carried away, it was easy to imagine an endpoint of inexpressible disaster.

But tuberculosis didn't bring an end to civilization. In fact, the battle against the disease ultimately demonstrated something quite different: human adaptability and resilience. This plague, the worst the species had known, brought out the best the world's greatest scientific minds had to offer. The medical profession rose to the challenge, joined together, and began the pivotal research that led to the cure for a seemingly incurable disease.

After all, desperate times call for desperate measures.

Robert Koch's Great Discovery

The road to find a cure for tuberculosis was a bumpy one. The first "bump" to be overcome was that no one knew what caused the disease. Despite brilliant research by Louis Pasteur, Joseph Lister, and others who demonstrated that microscopic organisms ("germs") might cause disease, the possibility that such a cause might exist for tuberculosis was long dismissed by experts. Up to the day that a young German physician and scientist named Robert Koch stepped up to deliver an address to the Physiological Society in Berlin on March 24, 1882, leading scientists still believed that inherited predispositions, sickly constitutions, or the body's own inflammatory poisons were to blame.

In undertaking his research, Koch came up with what are now known as Koch's Postulates, a brilliant and far-sighted set of rules designed to prove when a specific organism was the cause of a disease. To reach that conclusion, a researcher had to be certain:

- That the organism could be discoverable in every instance of the disease;
- That, extracted from the body, the germ could be produced in a pure culture, maintainable over several microbial generations;

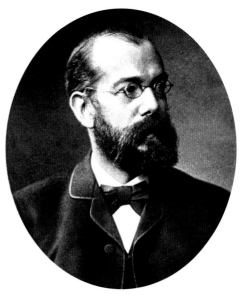

The face of a genius. The leading medical experts scoffed when a little-known physician named Robert Koch revealed that he'd discovered the pathogen that caused tuberculosis: a bacillus he named *Mycobacterium tuberculosis*. But the 1882 meeting in which Koch announced his discovery turned out to be a pivotal moment in the battle against the epidemic disease.

- That the disease could be reproduced in experimental animals
  through a pure culture removed by numerous generations from
  the organisms initially isolated;
- That the organism could be retrieved from the inoculated animal
  and cultured anew.

Having developed these postulates to study tuberculosis, Koch stepped
on stage to tell the august audience that virtually everything they thought
they knew about the disease was wrong. In an address that future Nobel
laureate Paul Ehrlich called "the most important experience of my scientific
life," Koch, a halting, mumbling man of little scientific renown, clearly and
carefully laid out his proof that the cause of tuberculosis was, in fact, a
germ—specifically, a previously unknown bacillus: *Mycobacterium tuberculosis*.

Knowing the skepticism with which his findings might be received,
Koch had brought his entire laboratory with him: microscopes, slides,
stains, test-tube cultures, tissue samples. He wanted no doubt to exist that
his findings were backed by hard science, especially since, as he said in
the lecture, "Those staining methods which have been so useful in the
demonstration of pathogenic microorganisms in other diseases have been
unsuccessful here. Every experiment devised for the isolation and culture
of the tuberculosis infective agent has also failed."

To an audience struck dumb by his claims, Koch described the
methodical analysis of his experiments. He showed tissue dissections from
guinea pigs that had been infected with tuberculous material taken
from infected apes, from the brains and lungs of humans who had
died from tuberculosis, from the inflammatory "cheesy" masses found
in tubercular lungs, and from the abdominal cavities of infected
cows. Again and again, he had found the tubercle bacteria in the
tissues of the infected guinea pigs—and in all cases, bacterial
cultures showed that the tubercles were identical.

"All these facts taken together can lead to only one
conclusion: that the bacilli which are present in the tuberculosis
substances not only accompany the tuberculous process, but are the
cause of it," Koch said. But he knew full well, as he watched the
eminent Rudolf Virchow storm from the room, that a long, painful
battle remained ahead before others were convinced.

Treatment: False Starts, False Hopes

Koch's lecture caused an immediate worldwide sensation. An editorial
in the *London Times* proclaimed, "If Dr. Koch's investigations and
conclusions should be confirmed by further experiments, we shall be
able to entertain a reasonable hope that an antidote to consumption

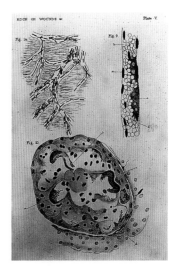

Robert Koch shared many characteristics
with the greatest scientists in history,
including a relentless determination to solve
medicine's mysteries and firm belief in his
ability to do so. Koch's scientific illustra-
tions, including this one showing bacteria
found in wounds, demonstrate his rigorous
precision and accuracy.

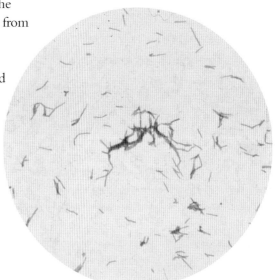

An image similar to what Robert Koch
would have presented in 1882: the bacillus
Mycobacterium tuberculosis. The stringy
clumping of the bacteria is called cording
and is found more frequently in *M. tuberculosis* than the nontuberculous mycobacteria.

and to tuberculous diseases generally may at no distant date be brought within our reach."

But Virchow was far from alone in denouncing Koch's findings and years passed before other experts lined up behind his theory. Textbooks published a decade or more after his isolation of *Mycobacterium tuberculosis* continued to trot out long-held beliefs about the cause of the disease, ranging from poor nutrition to "glandular enlargements." Koch's hypothesis was considered to be just one among many theories, conveniently ignoring the fact that the other theories were based on guesswork, and his was based on irrefutable science. It wasn't until the early 1890s that the general scientific establishment began to accept the truth.

At first, the fact that tuberculosis was caused by a bacterium only made its threat seem more dire. As the great physician William Osler estimated, a day's expectorations by a single patient might expel four billion or more bacilli, each capable of infecting a nearby individual—and each capable of wafting far and wide on the slightest breeze. How much more reassuring to believe in poor nutrition as the cause!

Despite the identification of *M. tuberculosis*, the fact remained that no effective treatment existed for this bacterial disease, and no one had any real idea of how to kill it. Yet that didn't stop so-called experts from hawking a wide variety of miracle cures and other panaceas. Advertised under homespun names like Mother Siegel's Curative Syrup and White Pine Compound, these mixtures differed in ingredients (cod-liver oil, various roots and leaves, herbs), but many of them made patients feel better by packing a strong alcoholic punch. None of them, of course, did anything to prevent tuberculosis's inexorable, destructive course.

Hopes flared briefly when Robert Koch himself announced that he'd devised a treatment for tuberculosis: tuberculin, a serum made from crushed *M. tuberculosis* (or the liquid it was cultured in) and administered by injection. In 1890 Koch announced that it provided an effective cure first in animal subjects, and then in humans with early forms of the disease. His announcement naturally caused a sensation, as patients with all stages of tuberculosis clamored for the treatment. Unfortunately, further testing revealed that tuberculin was ineffective in most (if not all) patients—though it remains in use today as a test to determine the presence of *M. tuberculosis*.

No miracle cures existed. There was just one thing, though far less modern-seeming than the various potions and injections, that appeared to help some patients with tuberculosis: rest, if not a panacea, at least provided a patient's lungs with the time to regain some lost strength. And it seemed better if this rest took place far from the crowded, dirty city streets and buildings where the disease thrived.

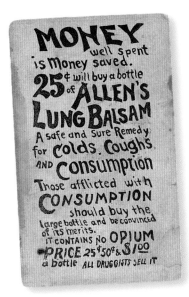

Purveyors of potions, salves, and other treatments reaped a rich harvest from desperate consumptive patients before the development of effective drug regimens. Many of these panaceas temporarily made the patient feel better—usually by administering a large percentage of alcohol— but did nothing to halt the spread of tuberculosis.

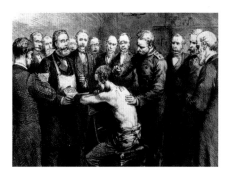

A nineteenth-century "inoculation" against consumption. For more than six decades after Robert Koch discovered the mycobacterial cause of tuberculosis in 1882, physicians remained unable to develop effective cures for the disease. Filling in the gap were countless useless treatments like this one.

Opposite: The mighty hero. Robert Koch portrayed as the new Saint George slaying the serpent of tuberculosis, after his 1882 discovery of the bacillus that caused the disease.

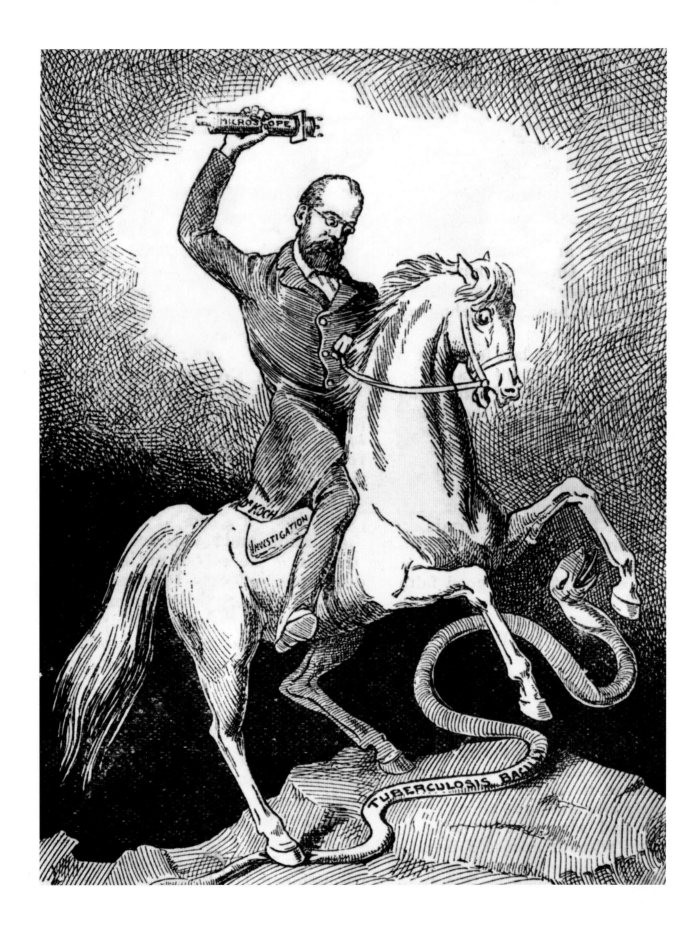

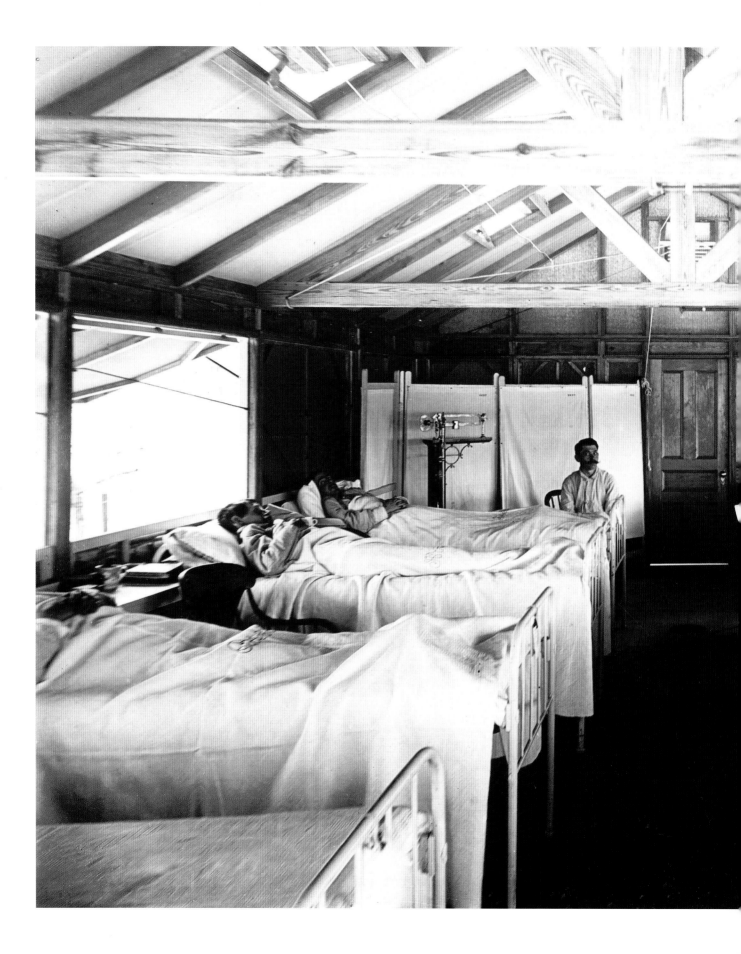

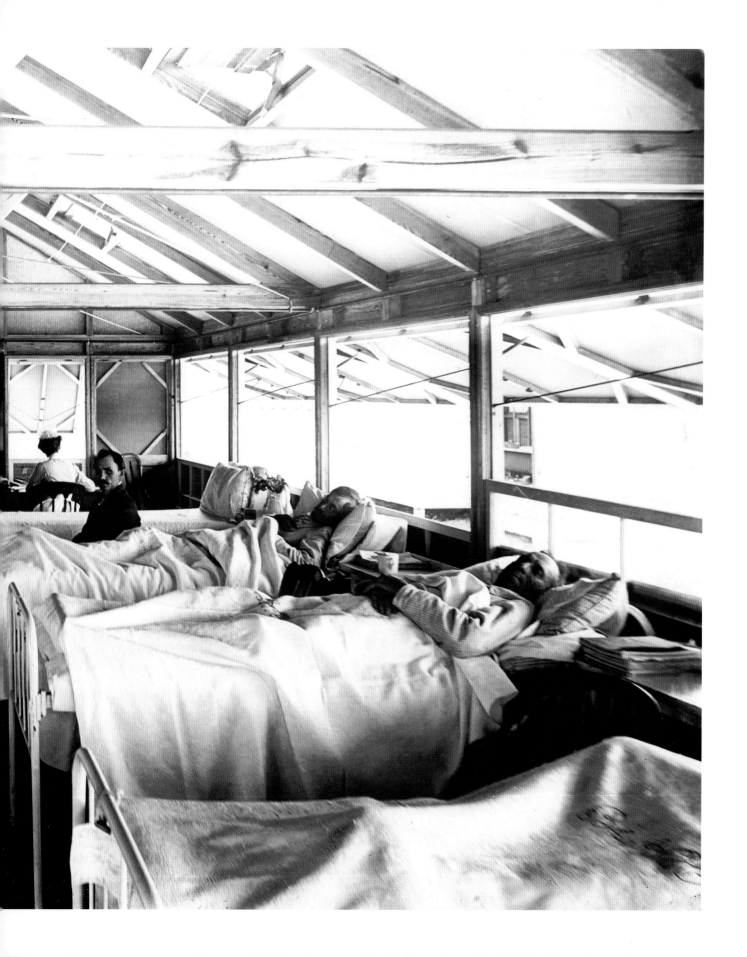

The Sanatorium Movement: "A Pure Atmosphere"

While it is obvious today that the crowded, airless, filthy conditions found in cities contributed greatly to the explosive spread of tuberculosis in the nineteenth century, few contemporary specialists paid heed. In fact, when a British country doctor named George Bodington decided that what sufferers needed was a "pure atmosphere, freely demonstrated without fear," no one much noticed.

In the 1850s, Bodington founded a small nursing home to provide calm, restful, open-air treatment to tuberculosis patients and unwittingly became the founder of a movement that would transform medicine for decades to come. This was the first sanatorium, the humble forerunner of the massive institutions that sprang up later in the nineteenth century, providing beds, healthful meals, and, above all, dignity, for tens of thousands of patients.

No credit was given to Bodington, however. When he published a book detailing his theories on tuberculosis treatment, he was excoriated by "expert" physicians. Forsaking his tuberculosis studies, Bodington spent the rest of his career studying and treating the mentally ill.

One physician did notice Bodington's innovative practices: Hermann Brehmer, who founded his own sanatorium in Germany in 1859. Located in the healthful mountain air, Brehmer's institution emphasized a healthy diet (including liberal doses of wine), careful exercise, and rest, providing the model for the sanatoriums to follow.

When a former patient of Brehmer's, Peter Dettweiler, opened his own sanatorium in Germany in 1876, the movement officially began. Within twenty years, sanatoriums sprang up across Europe. Some were tiny—just a rented house with a few beds and a small compound. Others catered to the poor and working class; these were often dirty and overcrowded, not much healthier than the grim tenements the patients had left behind. Still others were huge, sprawling estates, like the exclusive private sanatorium in Davos, Switzerland, immortalized in Thomas Mann's *The Magic Mountain.*

The United States and Canada soon followed the German model as well. Edward Livingston Trudeau, a physician and tuberculosis patient himself, learned of Brehmer and Dettweiler's efforts in 1882 and opened the Adirondack Cottage Sanitarium at Saranac Lake in New York. Starting out as just a smattering of houses and other small buildings, it grew to become the most famous sanatorium in the country. (While the words "sanatorium" and "sanitarium" were previously interchangeable, ultimately "sanitarium" referred to an institution used primarily for rest.) Dozens of others soon followed, many located in regions of the West and Southwest, where the dry air was considered to be especially healthy.

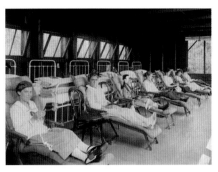

Many photographs from early sanatorium life showed patients lying in bed, but bed rest was not the only treatment: exercise and social interaction, though strictly regulated, were also important.

Previous spread: In the absence of effective medications, the best prescription for those with tuberculosis was often a visit to a sanatorium. Here, clean air, a mix of rest and exercise, nutritious food, and a variety of surgical procedures often led to improved health among patients.

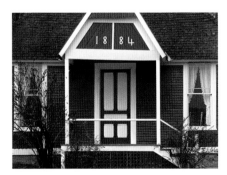

"Little Red," the small cottage built in the 1880s by Edward Livingston Trudeau in Saranac Lake, New York, that served as the United States' first tuberculosis sanatorium. Along with the Saranac Laboratory for the Study of Tuberculosis, the Adirondack Cottage Sanatorium (as Little Red and subsequent buildings were called) attracted hundreds of patients and dozens of doctors to the town, leading Saranac Lake to be dubbed "the city of the sick."

Edward Livingston Trudeau

THE PIONEER

Who we become so often depends on what we experienced as children. For Edward Livingston Trudeau, the child of a long line of physicians, a life spent working to help tuberculosis patients seemed fated almost from the start.

Trudeau was born in New York City in 1848. His first encounter with tuberculosis came early: before he reached the age of twenty, his older brother, James, contracted the disease, dying after just a few months.

While in college, Trudeau himself began to suffer symptoms of the disease, and by the time he was a young physician, pulmonary tuberculosis had put him on a downward spiral as well. To save his health, he moved his family to the Adirondack Mountains of New York, settling in the tiny town of Saranac Lake in 1876. Here he established a laboratory that soon became one of the most important centers for tuberculosis research in the world.

In Saranac Lake, Trudeau also brought to the United States a revolutionary European concept: the idea that tuberculosis patients might benefit from rest and exercise in clean accommodations amid a healthful rural atmosphere. In 1884 he opened the Adirondack Cottage Sanitarium, which within a few years became a sprawling mecca for tuberculosis patients. It was the first sanatorium built in North America, and inspiration for hundreds of others across the continent. Trudeau's motto was "To cure sometimes, to relieve often, and to comfort always."

In 1904 Trudeau was one of the founders—and first president—of the National Association for the Study and Prevention of Tuberculosis, the first incarnation of what became the American Lung Association. Though in frail health, in 1905 he also helped create the American Sanatorium Association, the organization that later became the American Thoracic Society.

Edward Livingston Trudeau died of complications from tuberculosis in 1915. He is remembered today by the annual awarding of the Edward Livingston Trudeau medal at the American Thoracic Society International Conference, given to the most

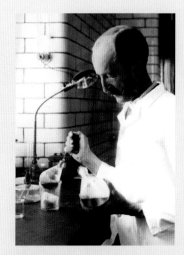

A visionary physician himself stricken by tuberculosis, Edward Livingston Trudeau brought both sanatorium culture and a laboratory dedicated to the eradication of the disease to tiny Saranac Lake, New York.

distinguished pulmonary scientists and physicians. In a celebration of his life and his sanatorium's twenty-fifth anniversary, Trudeau said, "Twenty-five years ago I dreamed a dream and lo, it has come true." His dream, and the determination with which he followed it, became a dream come true for those who found a better life under his care as well.

In addition to fresh air, extensive rest, and good nutrition, sanatoriums offered treatments ranging from hydrotherapy to phrenic nerve block. Lung support lay at the core of the Sanatorium Movement's program, and so surgeons also performed pneumothorax: the partial, controlled collapse of tubercular lungs to deprive the bacilli of oxygen and prevent their growth.

Sanatoriums also offered another benefit. As Frank Ryan points out in *The Forgotten Plague*, "The single most important achievement of such institutions—a very real and dramatically effective one—was the isolation of the infected from other potential victims." In addition, the rest and nutrition offered by the best sanatorium programs certainly made some patients' existence more tolerable, and may even have helped prolong their lives. But the truth remains that tuberculosis is a disease that does not often get better on its own, regardless of the quantities of fresh air and good food applied.

So was the great Sanatorium Movement merely a sideshow, a way to pass the time before a truly effective treatment was found? Not at all. In fact, the movement was revolutionary, not for what it did for patients, but for its impact on twentieth-century medical research, public health, and education.

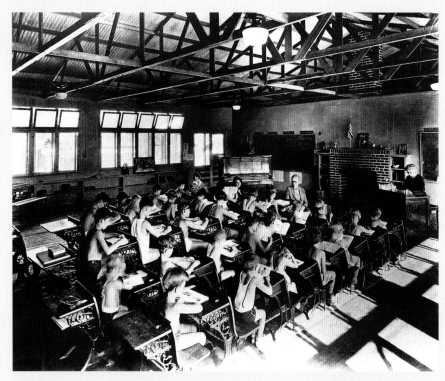

Just because you were living in the sanatorium didn't mean you got to skip school. In this 1910 photograph, young students attend open-air classes, dressed to take full advantage of the healthful country air.

Life in the Sanatorium

For patients wracked with the symptoms of pulmonary tuberculosis, spending time in a sanatorium must have seemed like the chance at a new lease on life. Many had spent their lives residing in smog-streaked urban neighborhoods, struggling through uncaring crowds, and working in airless factories. Many hated being a burden on equally overworked (and often, also ill) family members or friends. Who wouldn't have wanted to escape to the quiet, rural setting offered by most sanatoriums?

But sanatorium life wasn't the idyllic "month in the country" it is often portrayed as today, filled with long, leisurely walks alongside sun-dappled lakes and verdant, misty hillsides. Patients were expected to follow strict rules of rest, behavior, and social interaction. Posted schedules marked every minute of the day and forbade any deviation. As one sanatorium rulebook put it: "If you expect to get well you must work for it."

All patients were required to rise at the sound of the morning bell, often at first light. Since contemporary medical beliefs put great stock in fattening-up patients grown emaciated from the depredations of the disease, meals emphasized an abundance of dairy as well as other healthful foods such as eggs, steak, roast beef, bacon, game, baked potatoes, cauliflower, boiled spinach, a variety of other easily digested vegetables, and rice pudding or ice cream for dessert. Every meal had at least three courses, and many sanatoriums offered four such meals a day (along with nighttime snacks, if desired). Lights out was rarely later than 9:00 P.M.

Since both enforced rest and vigorous exercise were prescribed by tuberculosis specialists at the time, sanatoriums struggled to encompass these seemingly conflicting demands. Hours every day were spent in enforced bed rest, often with no talking allowed. On cold nights in northern sanatoriums, exercise and rest were combined in a way that patients sometimes found nightmarish: all but the most ill were required to undergo a form of "curing" that required sleeping on open-air porches in temperatures well below freezing. Instead, patients shivered sleeplessly through the night.

Occupational therapy, including crafts and other activities, filled the hours not spent in bed. At the Trudeau Sanatorium in Saranac Lake, New York,

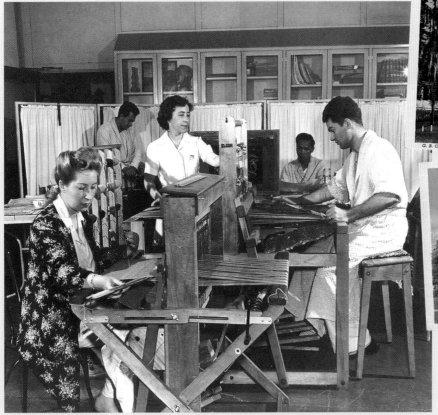

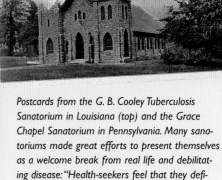

G. B. Cooley Tuberculosis Sanitorium, West Monroe, La.

GRACE CHAPEL, PENNA. STATE SANATORIUM, CRESSON, PA.

Postcards from the G. B. Cooley Tuberculosis Sanatorium in Louisiana (top) and the Grace Chapel Sanatorium in Pennsylvania. Many sanatoriums made great efforts to present themselves as a welcome break from real life and debilitating disease: "Health-seekers feel that they definitely 'belong' here, and that they are members of a community which understands them and takes them unto itself," proclaimed one sanatorium flyer.

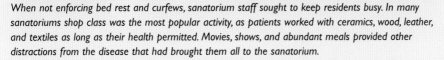

When not enforcing bed rest and curfews, sanatorium staff sought to keep residents busy. In many sanatoriums shop class was the most popular activity, as patients worked with ceramics, wood, leather, and textiles as long as their health permitted. Movies, shows, and abundant meals provided other distractions from the disease that had brought them all to the sanatorium.

patients could take classes in ceramics, woodwork, textiles, and other crafts. The actual objects produced by these classes—hand-painted shoe-trees, embroidered coat hangers and the like—were often useless, but the point was to fill the time in a healthy way.

Efforts were made to provide outside entertainment to patients at many sanatoriums. From early in the twentieth century, movies were always a popular choice—but the picture shows brought their own potential perils: Sanatoriums strongly discouraged socializing

between men and women and darkened movie theaters presented an obvious danger to the strict non-fraternization rules.

In response to the difficulty of enforcing such policies, some sanatoriums went so far as to regulate separate tables for men and women at mealtimes, and required them to maintain a distance of at least six feet from each other as they walked back to their cottages. Despite such rules—or perhaps because of them—every sanatorium saw its share of clandestine romances. Marriages of

sanatorium "alumni" were frequent as well.

Before they became ill, nearly every sanatorium resident would have laughed at the idea of submitting to such strict behavioral dictates. But in the age of the first tuberculosis epidemic, patients were willing to do anything to forestall the progress of their awful disease. They saw sanatorium life, despite its sometimes-cruel idiosyncrasies, as their last, best hope.

For the Public Good: The Creation of the National Tuberculosis Association and the American Sanatorium Association

Centuries of traditions dictated that the practice of medicine should be a solitary endeavor, but the tuberculosis epidemic clearly showed a team effort was needed to defeat the disease. In 1903 New York physician S. Adolphus Knopf called together the leading tuberculosis experts and succeeded in forming a committee of fifteen prominent medical figures, including Edward Livingston Trudeau, with the legendary John Hopkins physician William Osler as chairman. The committee's mission was clear: Twenty anti-tuberculosis societies had been formed before 1900, and they were to hammer out regional differences and form a national committee.

On June 6, 1904, in Atlantic City, New Jersey, the National Association for the Study and Prevention of Tuberculosis was formed. Later known as the American Lung Association, the association's members included both physicians and laymen, and Trudeau was its first president. It was the first national organization in the United States created to fight a specific disease, and was unique as well in its inclusion of laymen. Its goal was to be a model of organization and cooperation so powerful that it would bind together the laity, the medical profession, the state, and the nation in the common aim to defeat tuberculosis.

Raising money from wealthy benefactors such as John D. Rockefeller, the National Association almost immediately launched an education campaign to inform the public about the dangers of tuberculosis and the best ways to avoid contracting the disease. Public health programs taught citizens to cough into handkerchiefs and avoid infected people, and outlawed public spitting, among other things. At the same time, it lobbied state and local governments to build new sanatoriums and to establish public-health departments—another new concept at the time.

But the National Association was only the first national, cooperative group to form in the face of the ongoing tuberculosis epidemic. In 1905 Flick, Trudeau, and other National Association members with past or present involvement with sanatoriums met "to consider and, if deemed wise, to organize an association of men engaged in sanatorium work."

This made sense, since the physicians who founded, built, and ran sanatoriums faced challenges unknown to their colleagues. As Julius Lane Wilson, M.D., wrote in the American Thoracic Society's *American Review of Respiratory Medicine,* "These physicians staffed sanatoriums at isolated places in which they were not only responsible for the medical care of their patients . . . but also for administration; hiring and firing employees; supervising grounds and buildings, water supply, and sewage disposal; training assistants, nurses, and technicians and, most important, raising the

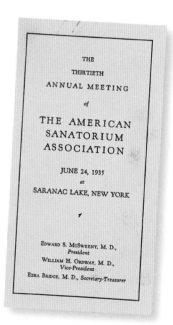

THE
THIRTIETH
ANNUAL MEETING
of
THE AMERICAN
SANATORIUM
ASSOCIATION

JUNE 24, 1935
at
SARANAC LAKE, NEW YORK

EDWARD S. McSWEENY, M. D.,
President
WILLIAM H. ORDWAY, M. D.,
Vice-President
EZRA BRIDGE, M. D., *Secretary-Treasurer*

A 1935 meeting schedule for the American Sanatorium Association, eventually to be renamed the American Thoracic Society. Started in 1905 specifically to address the needs of sanatorium directors, the Association soon expanded to embrace research and education into the causes and treatments of tuberculosis.

funds for operation and expansion from either private sources or state legislatures."

In 1905 this subset of physician/administrators within the National Association founded the American Sanatorium Association, which required participation in active sanatorium work and membership in the National Association from all members. By 1917 the Sanatorium Association had begun to publish its own journal—the *American Review of Tuberculosis*—carrying articles on the classification of the disease, diagnostic standards, and other crucial yet too-often neglected issues.

In the years to follow, the journal was renamed to reflect the Sanatorium Association's ever-expanding mission; first, the *American Review of Tuberculosis and Pulmonary Disease*, then the *American Review of Respiratory Disease*, and finally the *American Journal of Respiratory and Critical Care Medicine*. Today this publication, in conjunction with the American Thoracic Society's other journals, the *American Journal of Respiratory Cell and Molecular Biology* and *Proceedings of the American Thoracic Society*, play the same critical educational role for respiratory specialists that the *American Review of Tuberculosis* did nearly ninety years ago.

The Sanatorium Association renamed itself the American Trudeau Society in 1938, and then the American Thoracic Society in 1960, to reinforce its growing influence and scope. Though it started out specifically to bring national standards to sanatoriums, tuberculosis nomenclature, and other issues, soon the Sanatorium Association was focusing on important research into treatments for tuberculosis and eventually other respiratory diseases—the mission that, under its current name, it maintains today.

A Miracle from the Soil

Sanatoriums provided rest for the tuberculosis patient, but what was needed was a cure. The medical establishment agreed that tuberculosis was caused by a microorganism, but no one knew where to find something that could kill *M. tuberculosis.*

Soil microbiologist Selman Waksman finally discovered the solution: the cure to deadliest disease on earth lay in the earth itself.

The reasoning behind Waksman's supposition was sound, even profound. In an article (co-written with H. B. Woodruff) in *The Journal of Bacteriology,* he pointed out that disease-causing bacteria should exist in soil in great numbers, returned to the soil either in excreta or in the remains of their animal hosts. But it wasn't so. Waksman believed that the bacteria weren't there for a simple reason: because something as yet undiscovered had killed them. He suggested that, "the cause of the disappearance of these disease-producing organisms in the soil is to be looked

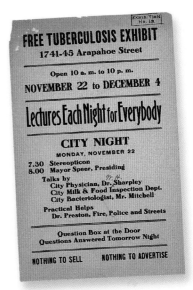

A flyer for a 1909 tuberculosis lecture. Tuberculosis was never far from the public's mind and lacking better alternatives, physicians and other health experts did what they could to educate the public on how to slow the epidemic's spread.

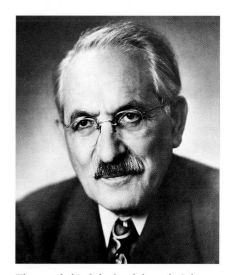

The man behind the breakthrough: Selman A. Waksman, Ph.D. Remarkably, it was Waksman, a soil microbiologist, who did what generations of tuberculosis experts had failed to do: find a substance that could not only halt the spread of tuberculosis, but eradicate *M. tuberculosis* within the human body.

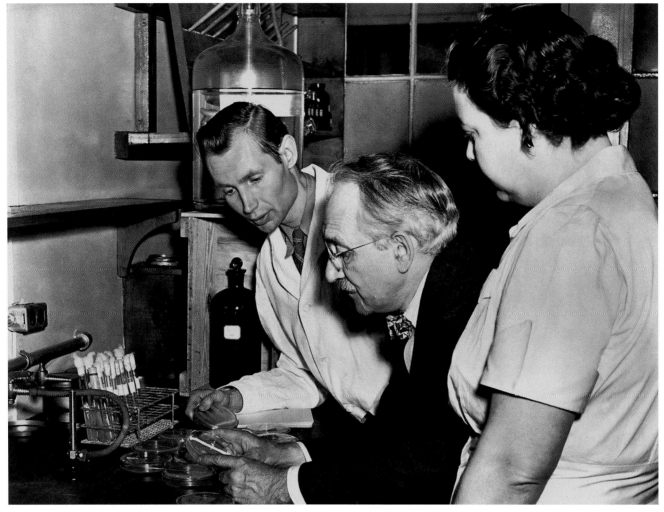

for among the soil-producing microbes, antagonistic to the pathogens and bringing about their rapid destruction in the soil."

Other researchers were close on Waksman's tail, and it was soon apparent to all that the soil was, in fact, fertile ground for antibacterial compounds. Early in the 1940s, the work of Waksman and his group produced antibiotics such as actinomycin and streptothricin that, while effective against bacteria, had unacceptably toxic side effects. These findings tended to confirm what naysayers had been claiming for decades about antibiotics: that most of those effective against disease would also be harmful to the patient.

But Waksman's team didn't give up. In 1943 he turned his attention to *Streptomyces griseus,* and soon found that it produced a substance he called streptomycin. In a table accompanying a paper published in January 1944, he and his co-authors detailed the dramatic effectiveness of streptomycin against a broad range of bacteria, including *B. mycoides, S. aureus, E. coli,* . . . and *M. tuberculosis.*

But, as Julius Comroe, Jr., described his *Retrospectroscope* article, "The word 'streptomycin' is in the table, the words '*M. tuberculosis*' are also there, and the tenth line shows that streptomycin was an effective antibiotic

Rutgers University graduate students look on as Selman Waksman examines the antibiotic activity of actinomycetes, microbes that live in the soil. It was one of those microbes, *Streptomyces griseus,* that led to the development of streptomycin, the first effective medicine against tuberculosis.

against the tubercle bacillus. But nowhere else in the article (title, introduction, discussion, or summary) are the words tubercle bacillus or 'tuberculosis' mentioned again. The death of the 'Captain of the Men of Death' came to the world unannounced!"

Waksman had made a great discovery—arguably the greatest leap forward in public health in the long history of medicine. But it took others to realize the importance of his discovery, to take that essential next step of turning an important laboratory finding into a treatment that would save the lives of millions.

The scientists who did so were a pair of researchers at the Mayo Clinic. They were William H. Feldman (a veterinarian) and H. Corwin Hinshaw, an M.D./Ph.D. in zoology. Working with scarce supplies of streptomycin provided to them by Waksman, the men began to test the substance on guinea pigs infected with virulent human tuberculosis. Midway through 1944, their initial supply ran out—but not before they found that the guinea pigs had tolerated streptomycin well, and that the drug had significantly reduced the disease's severity.

Now came the challenge of how to get more streptomycin to continue the testing. It was expensive and difficult to produce. If a new source couldn't be found, Feldman and Hinshaw might not be able to continue the tests, despite the early, promising results. The two researchers infected a host of guinea pigs in the hope that, if they got their hands on more of the drug, they would have subjects to test it on.

Not for the first time, Selmen Waksman had a brilliant idea. He was already working with Merck and Company, the New Jersey–based drug firm, and now he called the company and requested a meeting. Officials at Merck agreed, and Waksman showed up with Feldman and Hinshaw. Together, they asked the Merck officials to make more of the drug for their studies. The company's owner and director, George Merck, gave the go-ahead, though as a businessman he wanted something in return: Feldman and Hinshaw had to test streptothricin as well.

Merck did more than simply allow the development of the drug that was finally able to contend effectively with tuberculosis. He ordered fifty scientists associated with his company to study streptomycin, ensuring that, if proven effective, it would be publicly available as soon as possible. In 1945, as research and development of streptomycin intensified, Merck did something even more remarkable: at a cost of untold millions of dollars to his company, he returned the patents for the drug to Rutgers University so work on the drug could proceed unfettered.

Thanks to Merck and Company, both Waksman's continuing laboratory work and Feldman and Hinshaw's guinea pig study provided stunning results. In animals, at least, this drug was spectacularly effective. The next step was to test it on human subjects.

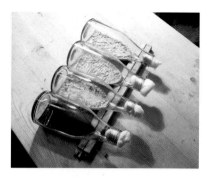

At long last, a weapon that worked. These vials contained cultures of *Streptomyces griseus*, the soil microbe. After fourteen days, the cultures produced streptomycin, a substance effective against bacteria in the soil—and also against tuberculosis and other diseases in the human body.

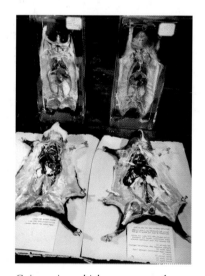

Guinea pigs, which can serve as host to virulent strains of human tuberculosis, played a huge role in the development of streptomycin. The first sign that the drug not only reduced disease severity, but was also well tolerated, came in animal studies involving these guinea pigs.

The first patients to receive streptomycin were an elderly man with tubercular meningitis in Rochester, New York, and a young woman in the last stages of pulmonary tuberculosis in Minnesota's Mineral Springs Sanatorium. The results were as dramatic, and as thrilling, as any researcher could ever imagine.

The elderly man died of an embolism, but postmortem revealed that the tuberculosis had been virtually extirpated from his body. The woman's case was even more encouraging: moved from the sanatorium to the Mayo Clinic because of the drastic worsening of her condition, she was close to death when streptomycin was administered. The drug's battle against the entrenched disease was a long one, but after months of treatment she was, by all clinical signs, cured.

Studies of greater numbers of individuals confirmed the results of these two cases. The first study, under the auspices of the American Trudeau Society, the precursor to the American Thoracic Society, combined data from several researchers who treated 332 patients. Of these, 86 percent showed clinical improvement, and in 82 percent, X-rays showed clearing. Further controlled studies produced equally impressive findings. But despite all the encouraging results from the early streptomycin tests, there were some disturbing signs as well.

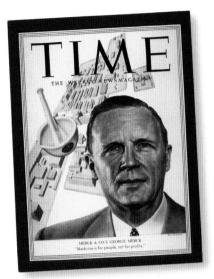

A *Time* cover featuring George Merck, founder of the great pharmaceutical company. Merck was an unsung hero of the quest to find an anti-tuberculosis drug, providing Selmen Waksman and his team of researchers with supplies of streptomycin to test on infected guinea pigs and then on human subjects.

A Resilient Enemy

It should have come as no surprise that a disease as ancient, as adaptable, and as easily spread as tuberculosis would not melt away in the face of the first effective treatment. As Julius Comroe said, "Streptomycin was absolutely essential in the therapeutic march against tuberculosis because it demolished the paralyzing concept that *nothing* would ever tame or kill tubercle bacilli in humans. But it was not a perfect drug. . . ."

It had, for example, some side effects, including damage to cranial nerves that could cause impairment in hearing or balance. More important, within a few years of its widespread introduction, it became obvious that certain strains of *M. tuberculosis* were developing a resistance to streptomycin. Patients who seemed to have been cured began to relapse.

Fortunately, the development of new weapons against the disease were not as long in coming as streptomycin had been. In 1940, a Swedish researcher named Jörgen Lehmann designed a substance that would interfere with the tubercle bacillus's biochemical processes. The result was para-aminosalicylic acid, or PAS. Alone, PAS was not a powerful weapon against tuberculosis, but in combination with streptomycin unleashed a more devastating attack on the bacillus than either drug did independently. Thus, physicians and scientists, near the dawn of the age of antibiotics, began to realize the utility of drug "cocktails"—a concept still in use today.

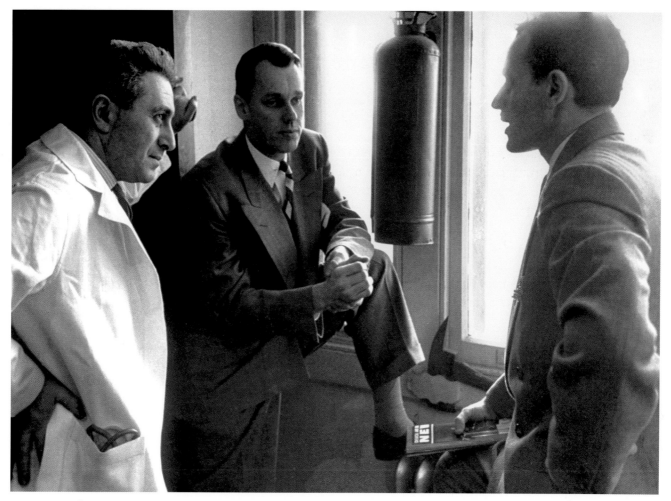

Another arrow in the quiver appeared in the early 1950s, with the arrival of isoniazid. The substance was actually first developed in 1912, only to be rediscovered decades later as perhaps the strongest drug against tuberculosis yet found. Isoniazid was followed by other effective drugs, including pyrazinamide, cycloserine, ethambutol, and rifampin. Countless patients were saved by use of these and other drugs, alone or in combination. With startling rapidity, tuberculosis went from being the dreaded white plague to a virtually forgotten disease in most Western countries, as much a part of the past as smallpox and the bubonic plague.

However, in the 1950s, after the disease's epidemiology had become far clearer, and after the armament of antimycobacterial drugs was well established, the annual death rate from tuberculosis worldwide remained at an astonishing five million people. The problem was not a lack of understanding or effective medications—it was the ease of spread of the disease and the difficulty of identifying, diagnosing, and treating infected patients.

In the mid-1950s, a team of researchers led by Richard Riley, M.D., of Johns Hopkins University proved William F. Wells's theory that airborne diseases could be transmitted via "droplet nuclei"—minuscule droplets containing one to three bacilli. Utilizing patients in a tuberculosis ward at

Isoniazid, first developed in 1912, became a vitally important weapon against tuberculosis in the 1950s, when Drs. Edward Robitzek (center) and Irving J. Selikoff (right) found that it was perhaps the most potent antimycobacterial drug yet discovered.

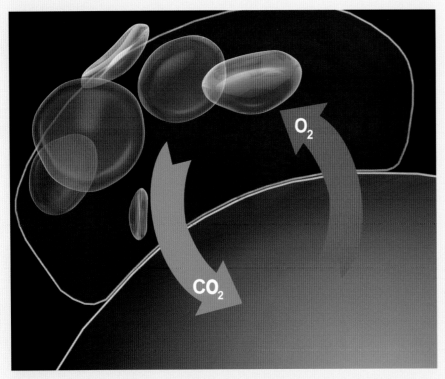

An image of gas exchange: the lungs diffuse oxygen to the capillaries through the thin walls of the alveoli, and the capillaries release carbon dioxide into the alveoli.

The Great Oxygen Debate

Discoveries in science often involve detours, missed opportunities, and outright mistakes before the truth in all its complexity is revealed. But rarely has there been a longer-running controversy, involving more famous figures in scientific history, than the decades-long debate over how the lungs release oxygen.

It was the French scientist Jean Baptiste Biot, studying fish swim bladders early in the nineteenth century, who noted that the bladders had a high concentration of oxygen, and concluded that oxygen

was being secreted. Since the swim bladder, like the lung, is a diverticulum of the gut, it was a logical step to believe that mammalian lungs must also secrete oxygen. Later in the nineteenth century, the German scientists Eduard Pfluger and Carl Ludwig simultaneously (and competitively) developed blood-gas pumps to look at the relationships between partial pressure and gas concentrations. Their findings inflamed the controversy, with Pfluger claiming that all gas exchange could be accounted for by diffusion alone and accusing

Ludwig of espousing the opposite despite the weight of the evidence.

John Scott Haldane, another giant in the field, sought to settle the debate. In the 1890s, Haldane developed his own device to measure gas exchange. His conclusion: "Absorption of oxygen by the lungs…cannot be explained by diffusion alone."

As it turned out, Haldane had committed several errors in developing his calculations. Further studies by him and Claude Douglas in the early 1900s came up with a different conclusion: the lung did not secrete oxygen under resting conditions, but did during muscular work, when inspiring a low-oxygen mixture, and during carbon monoxide poisoning. But the matter didn't rest there. Haldane's own son, the eminent biologist J. B. S. Haldane, undertook a series of studies that indicated diffusion was at work.

The final nails in the coffin of the oxygen-secretion hypothesis came from August and Marie Krogh, whose careful studies in the first decade of the twentieth century revealed that passive diffusion was the accurate hypothesis. The renowned Irish scientist Joseph Barcroft also came to the same conclusions around 1920.

By the 1920s the views of Barcroft, the Kroghs, the younger Haldane, and many others held sway. Except for a few remaining holdouts, a controversy that had spanned nearly a century had at last reached its conclusion.

a Baltimore Veterans Administration hospital, the researchers proved that guinea pigs could be infected simply by exposure to the air from the rooms containing the tuberculosis patients.

This knowledge of droplet nuclei allowed for a deeper understanding of how tuberculosis spreads. Scientists now know that one cough can contain as many as three thousand droplet nuclei, which are so small that they can remain suspended in the air for extended periods of time. The smallest can be inhaled deep within the lungs, finally lodging in the alveoli. Here they may be destroyed or encapsulated by the body's defenses, or they may begin to multiply, eventually converting to active disease.

The discovery of droplet nuclei as the mode of tuberculosis transmission also allowed physicians and scientists to discover that patients vary greatly in infectiousness; that infectiousness is greatly reduced with prompt, effective treatment; and that the average concentration of infectious droplet nuclei is low. All of these discoveries have allowed for the development of far more effective means to prevent disease transmission. Yet despite these advancements, tuberculosis is still a worldwide problem, one without a clear solution.

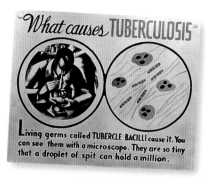

Before the development of effective anti-tuberculosis medications, the best weapon against spread of the disease was public information. This sign, posted at the 1936 World's Fair, would have been seen by thousands of passersby each day.

Tuberculosis: A Re-emerging Disease

In recent years, all of the advances in understanding, diagnosis, and treatment of tuberculosis—seemingly the keys to eradicating the disease—have met up with harsh reality. Half a century after tuberculosis slipped from the public's radar screen, the bald facts about the disease's continued prevalence are astounding:

- Currently, one-third of the world's population (about two billion people) is infected with the disease. Somewhere between 5 and 10 percent of infected individuals will develop active disease.
- Each year, about eight million people develop symptomatic tuberculosis.
- From 2000 to 2020 about one billion people become newly infected with tuberculosis. At least 200 million people will become sick from the disease, and thirty-five million will die.
- Tuberculosis and HIV are a particularly lethal combination. HIV promotes rapid progression of primary tuberculosis infection and is the strongest risk factor for reactivation of latent infection. Overall, one-third of people infected with HIV will develop tuberculosis.
- More women of reproductive age die of tuberculosis than of any other cause.
- More than a quarter of a million children die of the disease each year worldwide.

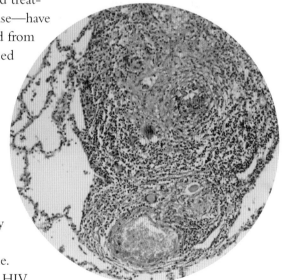

The tubercular lung. Today, physicians and scientists have access to medications, imaging technology, and other vital tools undreamed of a century ago. Yet in many parts of the world, tuberculosis continues to be a deadly epidemic disease.

Not surprisingly, the countries hardest hit by the resurgent tuberculosis epidemic are the ones least capable of managing accurate diagnosis and effective treatment. Three million new cases of tuberculosis occur each year in Southeast Asia; 1.5 million in sub-Saharan Africa; and millions more in Eastern Europe, especially Russia. Treatment for tuberculosis remains much as it has for half a century: a combination of familiar antibiotics, including the old standbys isoniazid and streptomycin. But, as author Lee B. Reichman, M.D., points out in his book *Timebomb,* "Paradoxically, although effective drugs and other interventions have been available for fifty years, there has been an embarrassingly meager effort to control the disease. We have the tools and we have not used them."

Admittedly, the challenge of confronting tuberculosis worldwide is a huge one, since the disease today cannot be cured with a quick course of antibiotic treatment. Instead, months of treatment with a complex drug regimen is required—a challenge for any individual, especially someone living in an area where health care is meager at best.

The World Health Organization has devised a program it calls DOT, for directly observed therapy, as the best way to ensure compliance. Though unquestionably effective, DOT requires political commitment, easily available microscopy services, dependable drug supplies, up-to-date surveillance and monitoring systems, and use of effective recommended regimes. Most important, a health-care worker must not only dispense medication directly to the patient, but also watch while the patient takes the medication.

The challenges are daunting. A 2003 update on tuberculosis treatment recommendations released by the American Thoracic Society, Centers for Disease Control and Prevention, and Infectious Diseases Society of America emphasized that DOT, to be successful, required such measures to facilitate adherence as "social support, housing assistance, coordination of tuberculosis services with those of other providers, referral for treatment of substance abuse, and treatment incentives and enablers."

In an admission of the difficulties inherent in such an approach, the report concluded on a sobering note: "The authors stress that the recommendations in their report are intended for treatment of tuberculosis in settings where mycobacterial cultures, radiological facilities, and drug susceptibility testing are available." In areas where these essentials are not available, the authors urge reliance on local tuberculosis control programs—assuming such programs exist.

It would be easy to despair at controlling tuberculosis even if every infected patient responded to treatment. During the past decade, however, the challenges have grown far greater as *M. tuberculosis,* already millions of years old, once again has begun to exact a fearsome toll—making it simultaneously one of the greatest medical success stories of the past century, and one of the greatest medical challenges of this one.

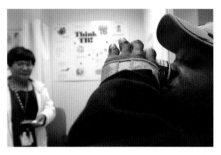

A crucial development in the treatment of modern-day tuberculosis is directly observed therapy. By watching as patients take their medicines, health-care workers (like this one in Newark, New Jersey, in 2002) can ensure patient compliance and help reduce the chance of outbreaks.

Opposite: Hilda Carrion, the first patient ever treated with isoniazid. Soon after the arrival of streptomycin, physicians began to see cases of drug resistance. Fortunately, a new array of drugs, including isoniazid, were quickly developed to augment streptomycin.

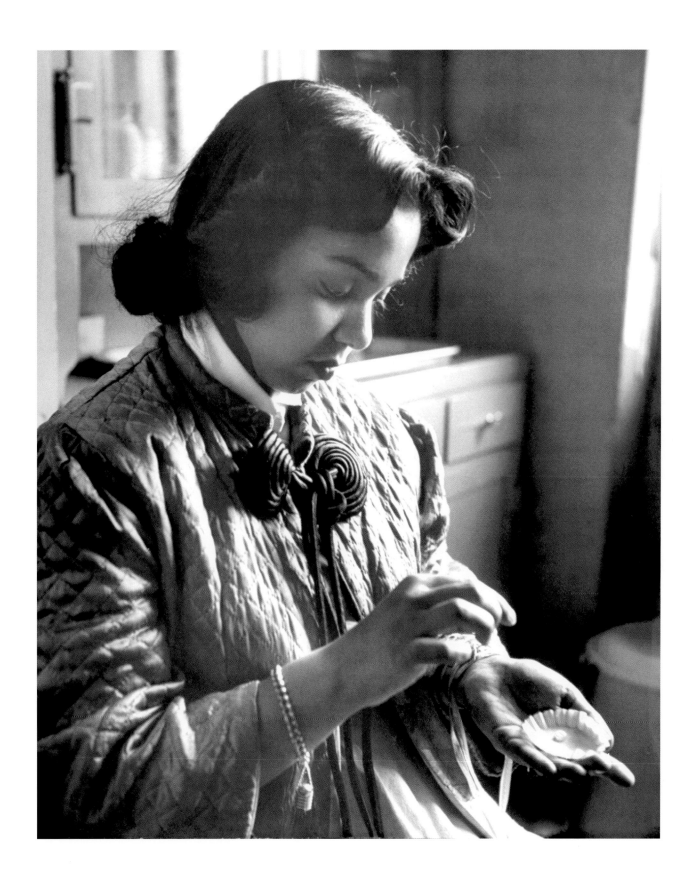

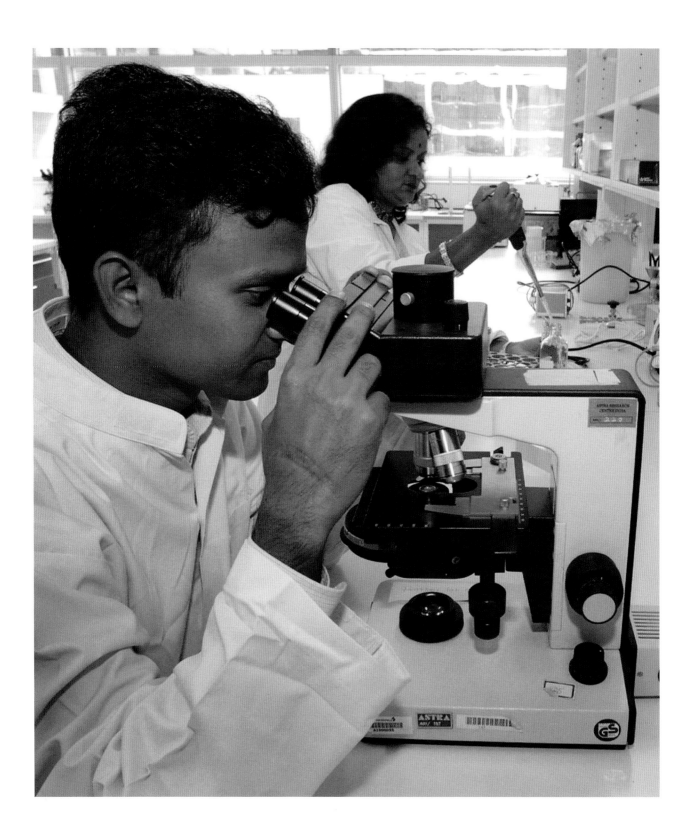

CHAPTER TWO

Broader Understanding, Broader Cooperation

"The only thing that will redeem mankind is cooperation."

—BERTRAND RUSSELL, LOGICIAN (1872–1970)

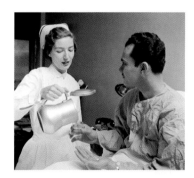

The heart of the issue: taking your medicine. When this tuberculosis patient received his doses of streptomycin, PAS, and isoniazid under a nurse's watchful eye in 1956, he was serving as a model for directly observed therapy, a vital aspect of the battles against tuberculosis today.

MEDICINE AS A DISCIPLINE grew to early maturity at the time of the tuberculosis epidemic—and in many ways in direct response to it. This era saw the development of anti-tuberculosis chemotherapy, the search for antibacterials in mold and in soil, and the use of carefully controlled studies to test treatments. However, these efforts were designed to combat tuberculosis, smallpox, syphilis, and a handful of other specific diseases, not to study the multitude of conditions that might affect the heart, the liver, or the lungs.

But as the twentieth century progressed, physicians and scientists alike sought a far deeper understanding of the body's organs and systems, and of the myriad diseases affecting them. With so many discoveries being made in so many different fields, it was imperative that everyone was able to share information. Local, state, and national health societies were pivotal in achieving cooperation across professions. The American Thoracic Society formed a natural link among physicians, patients, and the government, laying the groundwork for the medical research, public-health campaigns, and private-governmental partnerships that thrive today. Because of this link, the medical world was able to pass information accurately, share resources easily, and translate scientific advances into treatments quickly.

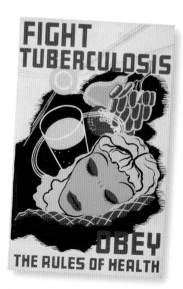

Just as Americans were warned to eat healthily and get plenty of rest back in 1940, public education continues to be a mainstay of the worldwide effort against respiratory diseases in the twenty-first century.

Opposite: A worldwide battle: scientists work at a new tuberculosis research facility in Bangalore, India, in 2003. Tuberculosis, like many other diseases, has global reach (two million new cases are diagnosed each year in India alone), requiring worldwide cooperation among physicians, scientists, and governments alike.

Expanding Roles in Pulmonary Health

When the National Association for the Study and Prevention of Tuberculosis was founded in 1904, its sole mission was to conquer that single dread epidemic. But something more was needed. Within a few

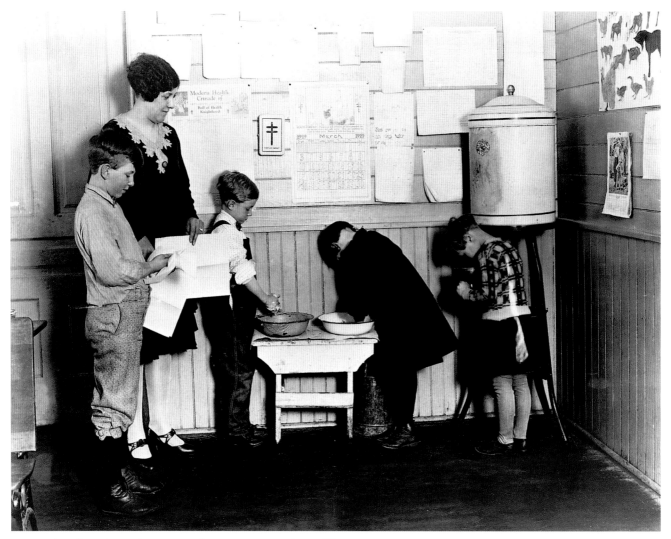

years of its founding, the National Association and its affiliated state associations realized that the structure of the organization and the enthusiasm of its members allowed for an expansion of the original charter. In 1917, the National Association's original program was altered to include children's health issues beyond tuberculosis. One early program was the Modern Health Crusade, designed to teach children about healthy diets, fresh air, and a number of other health-related issues. And beginning in 1924, affiliated organizations could attend to a wide range of other fields, ranging from heart disease and diabetes to cancer and psychiatric social work.

This widening of emphasis was not exclusive to the National Association. At the same time, similar issues were being debated within the American Trudeau Society, the precursor to the American Thoracic Society. The National Association mainly focused on public education and legislative work, and from the early years, the Sanatorium Association was widely viewed as the "scientific arm" of the National Association. This definition became official in 1915, when the Sanatorium Association was formally declared the medical section of the National Association.

While keeping your hands clean most likely did little to prevent the spread of tuberculosis, it certainly helped forestall the transmission of other diseases. Perhaps most important, education helped make the public aware that individuals could be responsible for keeping themselves healthy.

For at least two decades after its founding, the Sanatorium Association focused almost entirely on sanatorium issues and, more generally, tuberculosis treatment. In the 1920s, the focus changed dramatically as "collapse therapy" took hold among physicians treating pulmonary tuberculosis. The Sanatorium Association's meetings were first dominated by reports on artificial pneumothorax, then by more aggressive surgical approaches including phrenic nerve paralysis, thoracoplasty, plombage, and drainage of tuberculous cavities.

The arrival of surgery as an accepted—even embraced—method of treating respiratory diseases heralded the first stirrings of diversification within the Sanatorium Association. This diversification reached full flower when the organization settled on its current name, the American Thoracic Society, which reflects the Society's desire to work on all aspects of respiratory health associated with the "thoracic" or chest cavity.

Before this, however, in 1939 the Sanatorium Association changed its name to the American Trudeau Society. Its new constitution reaffirmed that tuberculosis would remain the primary purpose, and added "and related conditions" to the stated goals. Just as important, members would no longer have to be directly associated with sanatoriums. Chest disease specialists, general physicians, and those without a degree who had "attained special recognition in tuberculosis or other diseases of the chest" were all welcome. Under its new name, the American Trudeau Society truly had become a new organization. The question was how wide a net it should cast—whether it should be limited to conditions related to tuberculosis or should be concerned with other respiratory diseases as well.

In 1950 the Trudeau Society formed a committee to explore that question. But it wasn't until 1956 that the association's board of directors passed a resolution declaring that the charter would not be limited to diseases related to tuberculosis. The board pledged to make "the field of pulmonary disease an integral part of the program . . . and that this program should be extended to include the entire field of respiratory diseases."

Here, then, after many years and much debate, was the decision that determined the shape of the modern American Thoracic Society. The 1956 decision brought enormous change to the Society, whose new goal was to create a group of assemblies to confront challenges not dreamed of by the American Sanitorium Association's founders back in 1905.

Equally important was the consensus over who was needed to lead these new assemblies. "I can specifically remember Dr. William Tucker, one of the older and very well respected tuberculosis specialists of the day, making an impassioned plea to keep the old guys out of the leadership of these new assemblies," recalls William C. Bailey, M.D., in a piece written to celebrate the American Thoracic Society's centennial.

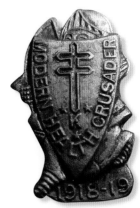

A "modern health crusader" pin circulated by the National Tuberculosis Association in 1918–19. At a time when a flu epidemic was sweeping the globe, the crusading efforts of private organizations and federal, state, and local health departments served crucial roles in slowing the spread of infectious diseases.

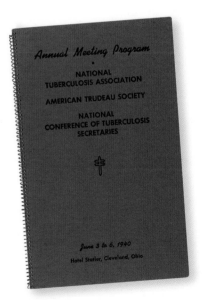

A program from the 1940 annual meeting of the National Tuberculosis Association (precursor to the American Lung Association) and its scientific section, the American Trudeau Society (forerunner of the American Thoracic Society). Together, the two organizations helped usher in a new age in medicine.

"He suggested that the ATS needed a whole new generation of leaders from fields that were, in many cases, in their infancy."

Today, the American Thoracic Society includes a dozen assemblies: Allergy, Immunology & Inflammation and its section on genetics and genomics; Behavioral Science; Clinical Problems; Critical Care; Environmental & Occupational Health and its section on terrorism and inhalation disasters; Microbiology, Tuberculosis & Pulmonary Infections; Nursing and its section on pulmonary rehabilitation; Pediatrics; Pulmonary Circulation; Respiratory Cell & Molecular Biology; Respiratory Neurobiology & Sleep; and Respiratory Structure & Function. Together, they make the American Thoracic Society more capable of confronting new challenges than ever before.

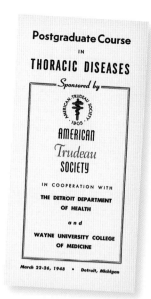

The American Trudeau Society offered this postgraduate course in thoracic diseases in 1948. Under its current name, the American Thoracic Society continues to play a central role in physician education, through its assemblies, grants, alliances with other organizations, and international conferences.

The National Institutes of Health

At the same time the American Thoracic Society was growing, the National Institutes of Health (NIH) were also expanding their reach. Founded in 1887, the NIH funded research into lung diseases, mechanical ventilation, and other topics relevant to respiratory medicine during its first three-quarters of a century. But it wasn't until 1969 that the NIH chose to officially welcome the respiratory system into its own system of Institutes, changing the name of the National Heart Institute into the National Heart and Lung Institute, and again to the National Heart, Lung and Blood Institute (NHLBI). The NHLBI also plunged further into another field: research.

In recent years, both the American Thoracic Society and the respiratory component of the NHLBI have sought a deeper understanding of how the lung functions at the organ, tissue, cellular, and molecular levels, while continuing to research the causes and treatments of pulmonary diseases. Under its Division of Lung Diseases, the NHLBI seeks answers to fundamental questions of lung cell and vascular biology, lung growth and development, pediatric lung disease, and other issues in the Lung Biology and Disease Program. Concurrently, its Airway Biology and Disease Program focuses on education and training in diseases including chronic obstructive pulmonary disease (COPD), asthma, bronchiolitis, and sleep disorders, as well as clinical and basic research.

Basic research has produced astounding advances in understanding and treating a variety of pulmonary diseases; results include the decoding of the human genome and the discovery of genetic bases for cystic fibrosis and other diseases. Equally important, however, has been a continuing emphasis on clinical research with a direct impact on patient care. These two fields of research combine in the NIH's Specialized Centers of Research (SCOR) program, unveiled in the 1960s to facilitate the translation of basic science to clinical practice. In addition, the NIH supports clinical pulmonary research

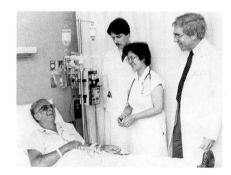

The National Institutes of Health (NIH) and its member institutes, such as the National Heart, Lung, and Blood Institute (NHLBI), have made an incalculable difference in improving our understanding of respiratory diseases. Here, a patient suffering from alpha-1 antitrypsin deficiency receives the first dose of Prolastin, the alpha-1 substitute, as NIH physician-scientists Ron Crystal, M.D., (standing right), Mark Wewers, M.D., (standing left) and nurse Peggy Leung (middle) look on.

through research project grants, career development awards, and Program Project Grants.

In the 1980s, the NIH, and its SCOR programs in particular, were facing budget cuts in Washington. It was time for the American Thoracic Society to step in.

The lung SCOR program directors—all of whom were American Thoracic Society members—began to work with their local lung associations to bring members of Congress in to look at the program. They came together in Washington, D.C., for a meeting that was set up and sponsored by the Rep. Al Gore, Jr.

The meeting was headed by Dr. Mildred Stallman, head of the Pediatric Pulmonary SCOR. As she entered the meeting room, she and the future Vice President Gore exchanged warm greetings. She then sat down and put two pounds of butter on the table in front of her and set up her first slide: a picture of a baby's hand on an adult thumbnail. "I save babies who weigh less than the butter in front of me," she told the representatives. "This slide shows Al Gore III and his father, Rep. Al Gore."

The impact of such a presentation was incalculable. Without question, this and other meetings organized by the American Thoracic Society contributed mightily to the rescue of the pulmonary SCOR programs from the budget axe.

Programs such as SCOR not only further specific kinds of research, they also further collegiality among researchers. It is this spirit of cooperation that has enabled many of the recent discoveries in lung physiology to come to fruition.

Pulmonary Partnerships:
Understanding Lung Structure and Function

The new spirit of camaraderie that organizations such as the NIH and the American Thoracic Society brought to the medical profession allowed physicians, scientists, physiologists, and other experts to begin to answer some of the basic questions that had confounded investigators for decades. Beginning in the middle of the twentieth century, a deeper understanding of lung structure and function finally developed.

One extremely important, though initially unlikely, team of specialists came together at the University of Rochester in New York under the leadership of Wallace Fenn, Ph.D. One member of the team, Hermann Rahn, Ph.D, was a specialist in frog hormones, while another, Arthur Otis, Ph.D, studied enzymes in grasshopper eggs. Putting aside previous interests to study gas exchange, they developed the oxygen–carbon-dioxide diagram, initially to analyze the effects of hyperventilation on alveolar gas composition at high altitude.

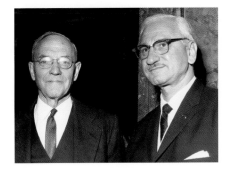

Professors Wallace Fenn (left) and Albert Sabin in Rome to receive awards from the Antonio Feltrinelli Foundation for Medicine in 1964. Sabin's award was largely due to his development of a polio vaccine, Fenn's for his outstanding work in pulmonary gas exchange and other findings that advanced scientific knowledge of lung structure and function.

The diagram, however, was extraordinary in its ability to take into account six variables: PO_2, PCO_2, respiratory exchange ratio, arterial oxygen saturation, alveolar ventilation, and barometric pressure (indicating altitude). The breadth of this accomplishment allowed investigators to study ventilation–perfusion relationships in great detail, and learn much more about abnormal gas exchange in diseased lungs.

At roughly the same time the Rochester group was making these strides, Richard Riley was following a similar trail in Florida. At the United States Naval School of Aviation Medicine, Riley worked with Joseph Lillienthal on a critical wartime problem: measuring carbon monoxide in the blood, in order to reduce the number of aircraft accidents caused by carbon monoxide poisoning.

In response to the wartime challenge, Riley designed the bubble technique for measuring partial pressures of oxygen and carbon dioxide in the blood, and used this knowledge to devise a method of understanding ventilation–perfusion inequality in diseased lungs, just as Wallace Fenn's group in Rochester had.

After the war, while confined to his home by pulmonary tuberculosis, Riley developed his model further. His analysis allowed for the division of the diseased lung into three compartments: the "ideal" compartment, which had optimal gas exchange; "dead space," which had unperfused by ventilated alveoli; and "the shunt," which had unventilated by perfused alveoli, concepts still clinically useful today.

These advances allowed researchers to understand disordered lung function more fully than ever before. But the three-compartment theory was at best a clumsy approximation of true distribution of ventilation–perfusion ratios in the lung. Not until the development of computer numerical analysis for studying the behavior of distributions by Kelman, West, Olszowka, and Farhi did scientists achieve a truer knowledge of ventilation–perfusion inequality.

While Fenn, Riley, and other researchers focused on gas exchange, still others focused on studying the lungs and heart under physiological conditions. While both at Bellevue Hospital in New York in the early 1930s, Dickinson Richards, M.D., and Andre Cournand, M.D., set out to prove, as Richards said after he and Cournand received the Nobel Prize in Physiology in 1956, "that lungs, heart, and circulation should be thought of as one single apparatus for the transfer of respiratory gases between outside atmosphere and working tissues."

The investigators determined that the only way to study pulmonary blood flow to their satisfaction was to devise a safe, effective method of catheterizing the heart. Overcoming the objections of those who thought that cardiac catheterization was neither safe nor feasible, they spent years designing and testing a method that successfully sampled

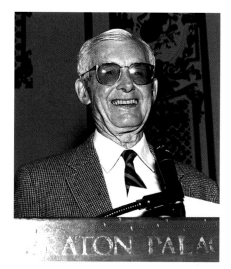

Richard Riley, a pioneer in untangling the mysteries of perfusion and ventilation in the lung. His division of the diseased lung into three compartments—ideal, dead space, and the shunt—remain in clinical use sixty years after Riley formulated it. Much of Riley's work in the 1940s was undertaken while he was confined to his home with pulmonary tuberculosis.

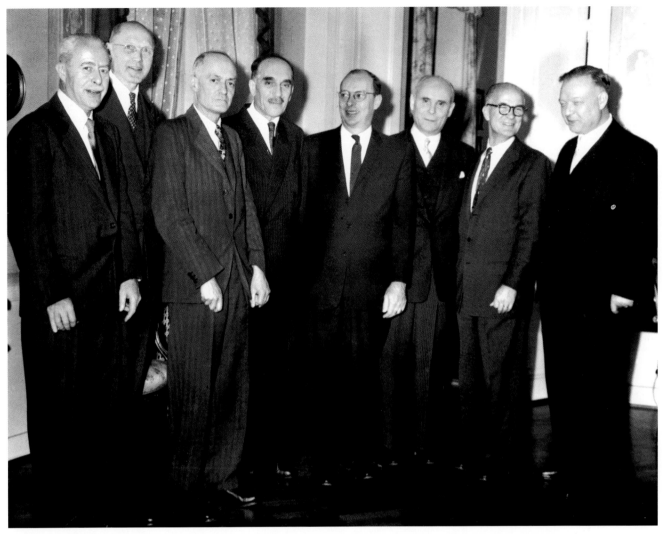

mixed venous blood and measured pulmonary blood flow. Their method, when applied to normal subjects, also allowed for an initial understanding of the hemodynamic abnormalities encountered in heart disease. Cournand's and Richards's proof that cardiac catheterization was not only feasible, but essential, led to their Nobel Prize.

Partnerships between doctors wasn't the only new development in collegiality: A classic example of joining disciplines for a single goal came in the work of a Swiss physician, professor, and anatomist named Ewald Weibel, M.D. Determined to untangle the complicated structure of the lung, Weibel decided to apply morphometric mathematical data analysis to the problem. Morphometry was first devised by geologists seeking a method to measure the volume of minerals in rocks, and allowed researchers to use a variety of samples from different experimental groups to recreate and study the three-dimensional structures present in the rocks. Weibel applied the same techniques to microscopic images of lung tissues and cells, and in the 1960s he created the most complete picture of lung structure available at the time, which remains in widespread application today.

A panoply of winners of the 1956 Nobel Prize. Included are Drs. Dickinson Richards (second from left) and Andre Cournand (third from right), whose brilliant work on right-heart catheterization and pulmonary heart disease opened new horizons in scientists' understanding of respiratory diseases.

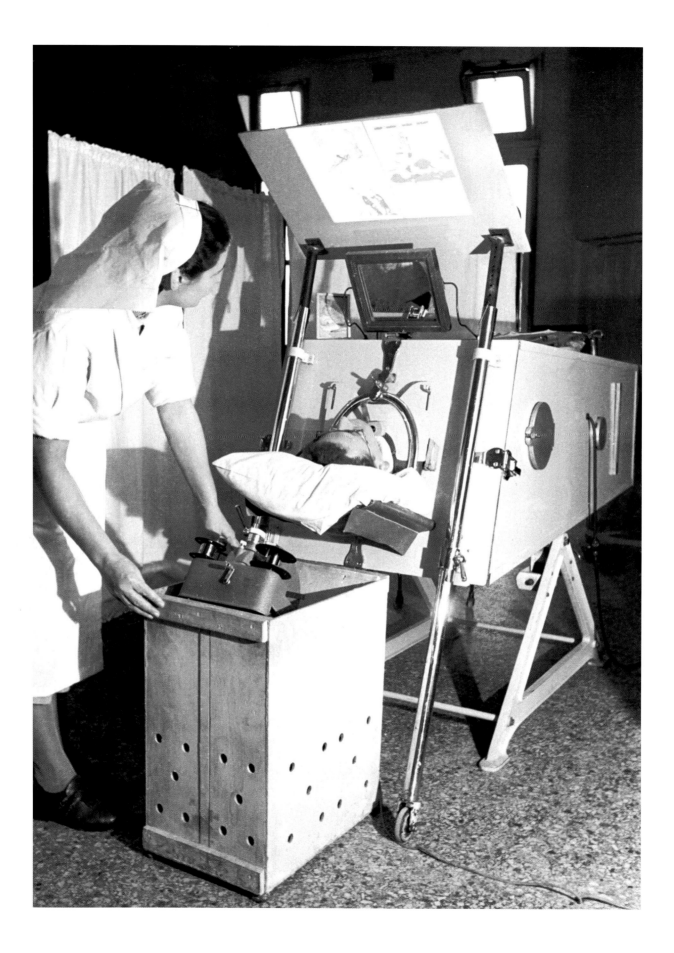

It is impossible to overestimate the importance of each of these advances. Along with many others, they provided essential platforms for decades of further research. But these crucial basic-science discoveries were just one side of the coin. In addition to learning about the structure and function of the lung, investigators sought to apply what they had learned to another crucial goal: to keep patients' lungs functioning.

The Iron Lung and Other Body Boxes

In an age when cures for tuberculosis, polio, and other diseases affecting the lungs remained elusive, the next best—and often only—option was support of patients' damaged lungs. Various body boxes have been designed to assist patients with breathing, and while most are obsolete, some are still in use today.

In 1885 J. Ketchum built his "pneumatic cabinet," a body box designed for a patient to either stand or lie down inside. The patient breathed through a mask and tube that led outside the box, while someone either pushed or pulled a rubber membrane covering an opening. A similar device was designed by O. W. Doe in 1889 for resuscitating infants: the entire baby except for the nose and lips was placed inside a small box, into which air was rhythmically blown and sucked back out.

The first true precursor of the iron lung—a device designed for long-term use in patients with polio—was unveiled by W. Steuart in 1918. In Steuart's device, which was designed for children, the child's head remained entirely outside the box, the rest of the child within it. A large bellows then pumped air into the box and pulled it out, the pressure changes causing the child's lungs to inflate and deflate.

None of these devices achieved widespread use. In 1929, however, Harvard Professor of Industrial Hygiene Philip Drinker, assisted by Louis Agassiz Shaw, came up with a "body box" that likely helped save thousands of lives in the following three decades.

Drinker and Shaw's research was first sponsored by New York's Consolidated Gas Company, which sought a way to treat respiratory failure caused by carbon monoxide poisoning. The researchers' solution, a portable iron chamber designed for both adults and children, turned out to be ideal for polio patients as well.

The Drinker-Shaw model was both utilitarian and more comfortable than previous

Opposite: A nurse projects the pages of a book for a patient confined to an iron lung in this 1949 photograph. Iron lungs saved the lives of thousands of patients stricken with polio before the development of the first polio vaccines.

In 1929 Harvard researcher Philip Drinker was enlisted by New York's Consolidated Gas Company to create a device to treat patients suffering from carbon monoxide poisoning. In addition, the iron lung designed by Drinker and his assistant, Louis Agassiz Shaw, kept alive thousands of polio patients who otherwise would have died.

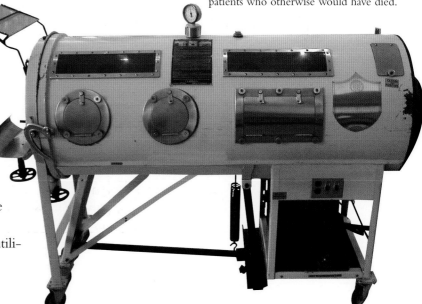

attempts. The patient's head was placed outside the chamber as in Steuart's box, with a rubber collar creating a seal by fitting snugly around the neck where it emerged from the box. A pair of vacuum pumps kept up a rhythmic push-pull motion on the chest, creating "breathing" in patients whose lungs were no longer able to draw in air for themselves.

The basic design of the Drinker-Shaw iron lung remained the industry standard through the repeated polio epidemics that occurred into the 1950s. Not that it remained unchanged, of course; modifications of the earliest, most cumbersome designs were inevitable. For example, the Both iron lung, first marketed by Both Equipment in 1938, was lighter and easier to use than the original, but its shape and wooden construction made it resemble a coffin, and it also lacked heating, lighting, or an alarm. These drawbacks led Captain G. T. Smith-Clarke, a former British auto executive, to unveil a new iron lung in the early 1950s.

The Smith-Clarke design was exactly what you'd expect from someone who'd spent his life around cars. This iron lung had large windows, strip lighting, a footrest, a tilting mechanism, wheels, and an alarm. It even had a hinged top (similar to a hood) that swung open for easy access to the interior, a feature that caused it to be dubbed the "alligator."

The 1950s also saw the widespread development of a less flashy, but far more important, advance in ventilation technology: positive-pressure ventilation. Earlier in the century, John Emerson, Alvin Barach, and others had experimented with positive pressure ventilation to treat patients with lung edema. Then, during World War II, Barach and others developed the first pneumatic valving systems to supply oxygen to high-altitude pilots, technological advances equally useful for anesthesia use and ventilatory support. These simple valving systems, when attached to a high-pressure gas source, soon became invaluable providers of life support in field hospitals worldwide.

But the true flowering of positive-pressure technology did not come until 1959, when J. M. Frumin demonstrated that an elevated positive end-expiratory pressure (PEEP) improved oxygenation in infiltrative lung disease. PEEP increases the volume of gas remaining in the lungs at the end of expiration, reducing the shunting of blood through the lungs and improving gas exchange. Frumin's critical finding confirmed that positive pressure could be used to prevent alveolar collapse (de-recruitment) at the end of a positive-pressure breath. Today, the importance of PEEP in maintaining gas exchange in diffuse lung injury is perhaps most tellingly demonstrated in the management of Acute Respiratory Distress Syndrome (ARDS).

The 1970s saw breakthroughs in both technology and in understanding that "non-physiologic" ventilatory patterns might benefit patients with severe respiratory failure. This decade saw the development of the idea that long inspiratory time patterns ("reverse ratio" ventilation) might

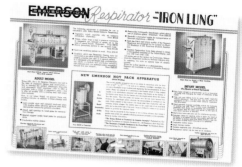

Polio made no distinction between young and old, and as a result iron lungs came in all sizes as well. Until the 1950s, fear of polio epidemics was widespread, and advertisements like this one were a common sight in many newspapers.

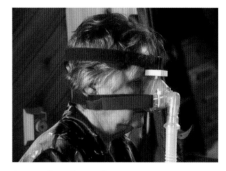

A great leap forward over negative-pressure devices, positive-pressure ventilation methods, including continuous positive airway pressure (CPAP), increase oxygenation to the lungs in patients who are breathing spontaneously, thus reducing the work of breathing.

Parker B. Francis

MEDICAL PHILANTHROPIST

As early as 1913, under the leadership of Parker B. Francis, the Kansas City Gas Company (later named Puritan) was specializing in delivery of compressed oxygen and nitrous oxide.

In 1940 Francis commissioned V. Ray Bennett to design gas-delivery devices for the company. Among Bennett's creations was the jeweled pneumatic flow valve. "The valve that breathes with the patient" was a design that spawned a series of innovative mechanical ventilators. The success of the joint enterprise led to a permanent partnership, the Puritan-Bennett Company, as well as a string of further successes in the development of respiratory equipment and medical gas delivery.

In 1951, recognizing the inextricable tie between his company's products and respiratory medicine, Parker B. Francis established a foundation bearing his name, with pulmonary research as its focus. Increases in Foundation resources led to the 1975 creation of the Parker B. Francis Fellowship program, a national postdoctoral fellowship training program in pulmonary research. In the thirty years since, according to current director Dr. Joseph P. Brain of the Harvard School of Public Health, the Francis Families Foundation has contributed more than $33 million to the Fellowship Program in support of more than five hundred Fellows.

"These talented Fellows have produced more than two thousand published works about lung biology and pulmonary research," Dr. Brain adds. "More importantly, these Fellows represent an entire cadre of physicians/scientists sprinkled throughout Canada and the United States, who are making a significant difference in the fight against lung disease."

A savvy businessman and generous philanthropist, Parker B. Francis and his

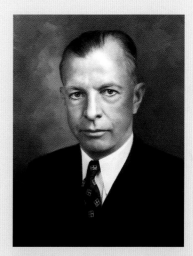

Parker B. Francis designed respiratory equipment and ventilators, but his greatest contribution was establishing the foundation that now bears his family's name, which has supported the research of hundreds of respiratory specialists.

Foundation recognized the need for widespread cooperation in the ongoing battle against respiratory disease and his substantial financial support continues his desire for cooperation to this day.

improve gas mixing and limit maximal airway pressures. In addition, the first commercially available high-frequency ventilators (HFV) were introduced. The non-convective gas transport mechanism of HFVs allowed for considerable lung recruitment but with low maximal pressures—a combination particularly beneficial in neonatal/pediatric patients at risk for overdistention injury.

In the 1980s, the use of mask positive-pressure systems achieved new importance. Continuous positive airway pressure (CPAP) is a method of positive-pressure ventilation used with patients who are breathing spontaneously, in which pressure in the airway is maintained above the level of atmospheric pressure throughout the respiratory cycle. The purpose is to keep the alveoli open at the end of expiration and thus increase oxygenation and reduce the work of breathing. CPAP, administered via tubes through a small mask or nose prongs, was found to provide effective non-invasive support for patients with obstructive sleep apnea and later for patients with acute obstructive airway disease.

The 1990s saw both the development of new innovations in positive-pressure ventilation technology (including harnessing the computer to ventilator systems) and a renewed interest in ventilator-induced lung

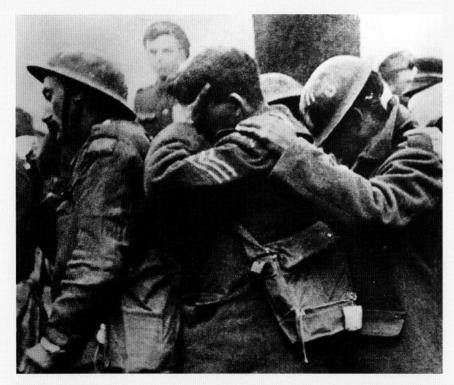

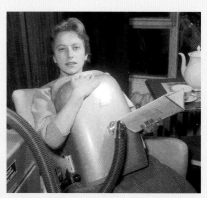

Advances in technology and the science of lung physiology during World War II allowed for the development of portable ventilators like the one above. Further refined in the late 1940s and early 1950s, these small machines have since saved thousands of lives.

World War I soldiers blinded by mustard gas, which also wreaked havoc on the lungs of those unfortunate enough to be exposed to it. Physicians treated as many as four hundred thousand victims of mustard gas during the war.

War and the Lung

Wars place extreme demands both on their combatants and also on the physicians treating them. By providing distressing new data on the effects of mustard, chlorine, and other gases on the lungs, World War I sped up the development of portable ventilators—an advance useful not only on the battlefield, but in peacetime conditions as well.

Despite the development of smaller, more portable means of supporting respiration during pulmonary surgery, World War I is best remembered for a more malign reason: it gave specialists a textbook

course in how various gases damage the lungs. While use of poison gas dates back to the mixture of wood, pitch, and sulfur set afire by the Spartans in war against Athens twenty-five hundred years ago, gas as a weapon was used most ferociously during the first World War. Mustard gas, the most lethal because it burns the lungs and eats away at exposed skin, is thought to have been responsible for as many as four hundred thousand casualties during the war.

By the end of the war, lung specialists knew more than they

wished about the clinical effects of these gases. While there is still no specific antidote for mustard gas, exposure can be avoided by wearing protective clothing and masks. There was, however, one unlikely benefit to come out of the horrors of mustard gas: it has been found to be an effective chemotherapy treatment for cancer victims.

Though the militaries of several countries continued to produce and study it, poison gas was not widely used in World War II. But this war, too, left its indelible imprint on the history of respiratory medicine, in

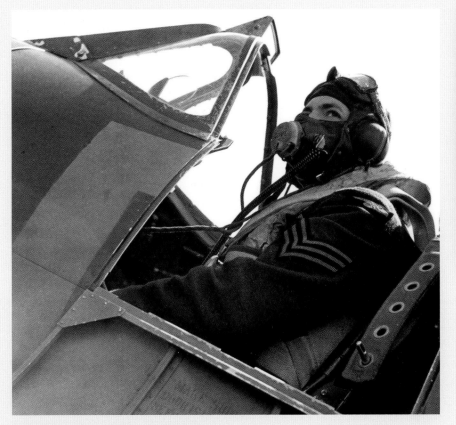

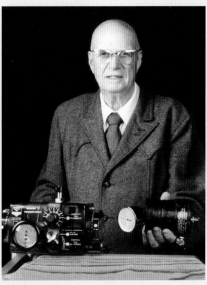

Forrest Bird, a technical air training officer in Army Air Corps during World War II, helped develop air-delivery systems to high-altitude pilots. After the war, he turned his attention to mechanical ventilation, and in 1954 unveiled the Bird Universal Mechanical Respirator, one of the first medical respirators.

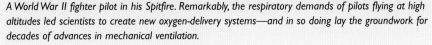

A World War II fighter pilot in his Spitfire. Remarkably, the respiratory demands of pilots flying at high altitudes led scientists to create new oxygen-delivery systems—and in so doing lay the groundwork for decades of advances in mechanical ventilation.

the form of extraordinary technological advances that helped lead to the modern age of mechanical ventilation.

As high-altitude fighter jets replaced biplanes and trench warfare in World War II, new demands were placed on the military personnel operating the new technologies. The most important question was how best to get enough oxygen into pilots' lungs to allow them to keep their heads clear and their reflexes sharp. Companies such as Lockheed and Sperry Gyroscope devoted

enormous time, money, and manpower to the task. In its laboratories on Long Island, New York, Sperry constructed a large "high-altitude room" that could vary its atmospheric pressure up to the equivalent of sixty thousand feet. One newspaper writer invited to inspect the room reported that the scientists moving about inside it "looked like Martians in their oxygen masks and electrically heated suits and boots," a stark indication of the harsh conditions high-altitude pilots operated under every time they flew. Intricate

masks were developed, enabling pilots to breathe easily and focus on the tasks at hand.

Inventors spent the wars trying to protect soldiers from toxic gases and improve upon the delivery systems of oxygen masks. In effect, they were pushing ahead advances in mechanical ventilation that otherwise might have taken years to perfect.

injury. Studies show that both underrecruitment and overdistention can produce lung injury, as well as the potential for the injured lung to release inflammatory cytokines into the circulation and cause multi-organ failure. In 1998 Amato reported significantly reduced mortality if ventilator management strategy was aimed at maximizing recruitment and minimizing end-inspiratory distention—a breakthrough finding particularly important in the management of ARDS.

Today, there are an estimated one hundred thousand positive-pressure ventilators in use worldwide. A deeper understanding of lung physiology and disease, the arrival of the computer age, and a myriad of advances in monitoring and ventilation technology mean that countless patients who would have died a generation ago now survive. However, mechanical ventilation did not solve all respiratory problems. In order to find cures for other diseases, further knowledge of the lung itself was crucial. One key to many diseases in the lung lay in a substance called surfactant.

The Secrets of Surfactant

Today surfactant is widely recognized as a fundamental part of lung development, yet until the 1950s, it wasn't even known to exist. The first step in the discovery of this vital fluid is credited to the Swiss physiologist Kurt von Neergaard.

Neergaard stumbled upon the theory for surfactant by studying lung elasticity, co-writing a paper on the subject in 1927. As he recalled his groundbreaking research, this early study provided him with some insights into the lungs that no earlier physiologists had ever gained. "The lung is probably unique among tissues in its extraordinary ability to expand and retract," he began in a paper in 1929. But, he went on, while most researchers believed that this ability was due solely to the elasticity of lung tissue, no study had demonstrated this. "So far," he pointed out in two of the most important sentences in the history of respiratory medicine, "one force has not been taken into account that definitely merits consideration. This is *surface tension*."

Neergaard did more than suggest the existence of surface tension at the boundary between the alveolar epithelium and alveolar air, and its crucial role in the expansion and retraction of the lungs. He went on to explain exactly how the process could work, even suggesting that some as-yet unidentified substance might cause the surface tension of alveoli to be lower than that of other body fluids. This lower tension, he explained, might be useful "because without it pulmonary retraction might become so great as to interfere with adequate expansion."

Looking back, it's clear that Neergaard, even if he was wrong in some details, had made a stunning conceptual leap. But a quarter century passed

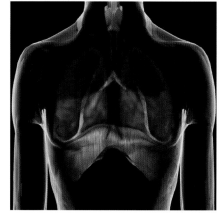

The respiratory system, a marvel of complex interaction between the outside world and the human body. War, disease, new technologies, and brilliant scientific research together have provided a deeper understanding of the respiratory system than could have been dreamed of a few generations ago—but much still remains to be learned.

before any follow-up investigations took place. Researchers instead focused on what they called "hyaline membranes," smooth material found in the lungs of newborns who had died following severe respiratory distress. The fact that such "membranes" were the result, not the cause, of severe respiratory distress didn't stop a generation of investigators from focusing on them.

The next true leap forward didn't occur until after World War II— and, as with so many advances in respiratory medicine, it was intimately connected with the war itself. Scientists Richard Pattle, M.D., and John Clements, M.D., were responsible, and the chemical warfare departments of the U.S. and British military supported their research after the war ended.

Richard Pattle made the first breakthrough in a way typical of evolutionary leaps in medicine: he was looking for something else. Assigned to find an antidote to phosgene gas, which kills by asphyxiation following pulmonary edema, Pattle instead discovered that the foamy fluid created by the edema seemed to be composed not of previously known components, but of some unidentified substance lining the surface of the alveoli. He also found that healthy lungs too created this mysterious substance—and that, importantly, the bubbles in this foam were remarkably stable, lasting for an hour or more, compared to just a few minutes for bubbles in blood and other fluids. Clearly, Pattle realized, the pulmonary foam must have extremely low surface tension.

Pattle's observations, published in *Nature* in 1955, piqued John Clements's curiosity. Clements, working at the Army Chemical Corps Medical Research Laboratory in Edgewood, Maryland, sought to find the correct measurement of pulmonary surface tension—and therefore pulmonary surface area. Building a modified surface-film balance which utilized a shallow trough equipped with a movable barrier at one end and a platinum strip attached to a force transducer at the other, Clements was able to make a series of remarkable discoveries about the still-unidentified fluid that lined the alveoli. He found that the fluid's surface tension was not only extraordinarily low, but varied greatly depending on surface area. When stretched out in the surface-film balance, it had a surface tension of 45 dynes/cm, but when compressed, the surface tension fell below 10 dynes/cm.

Clements, the first to understand the implications of the fluid, was also the first to give it the name "pulmonary surfactant." First of all, he explained, surfactant is what keeps the body's 300 million alveoli from collapsing under the pressure exerted within the lung. Further, when the lungs expand, the surface tension rises, keeping the lungs from overexpanding and helping them return to normal size. Finally, variations in surface tension depending on surface area allow alveoli of different sizes to function with equal efficiency in the healthy lung.

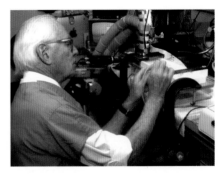

Dr. John Clements, a pioneer in the pediatric pulmonary field, has saved innumerable children with his discoveries about surfactant. Fifty years later, he is still researching the fluid.

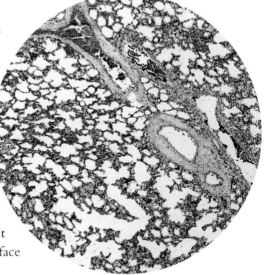

The lung of a healthy child. Breathing is effortlessly automatic in most children, as air enters the trachea and travels to the alveoli, where oxygen passes to the bloodstream and is exchanged for carbon dioxide.

Working separately but with a combined momentum little seen in previous respiratory research, Pattle and Clements had at last discovered the key to understanding how the lungs operated. What remained now was for someone to take their findings and apply them to real-world pulmonary diseases. That someone was a Harvard pediatrician and researcher named Mary Ellen Avery.

From the Bench to the Bedside: Mary Ellen Avery and NRDS

Avery was subsequently chief of Pediatrics at Harvard Medical School, physician-in-chief at Children's Hospital in Boston, and president of the American Association for the Advancement of Science. At the time of Pattle's and Clements's research, however, she was a young female physician starting out in a male-dominated field.

Avery's story is a famous one in the overall history of respiratory medicine. In 1952, soon after graduating from Johns Hopkins University School of Medicine, she contracted pulmonary tuberculosis. She stayed briefly in a sanatorium and then spent a year at her parent's home.

"During that time I corresponded with Richard Riley, my teacher at Johns Hopkins, about the rationale for bed rest; thus my quest for more knowledge of respiratory physiology began," she recalled in a 2000 article for the American Thoracic Society's *American Journal of Respiratory and Critical Care Medicine.* Her disease arrested and she was able to start her career: pediatrics with a subspecialty in pulmonary disease. "I was fortunate," she said, "to have been in the right place at the right time."

Every pediatrician in the 1950s was intimately familiar with the tragedy of what was then called "hyaline membrane disease." Now known as Neonatal Respiratory Distress Syndrome (NRDS), the leading cause of death among premature infants once claimed twenty thousand lives each year in the United States alone. But while its course was well known—NRDS usually occurs within four hours of birth and persistently worsens for forty-eight hours before either leading to death or resolving spontaneously—its causes remained a deep mystery until the 1950s.

At the time, experts still believed that the glassy hyaline membranes were in some way the cause of the often-fatal disease, speculating that they were composed of some substance that entered the newborn along with food, or arose from a viral infection. But these were just guesses. Avery wanted proof.

She underwent intensive training in advanced research techniques, funded by the National Institutes of Health (NIH), at Boston's Lying-In

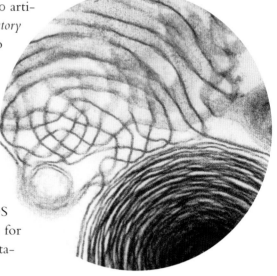

An electron micrograph of surfactant, a necessary substance in the lungs. Before Mary Ellen Avery, Jere Mead, and others identified the absence of surfactant in some premature babies, no one knew why twenty thousand babies died of suffocation each year soon after birth.

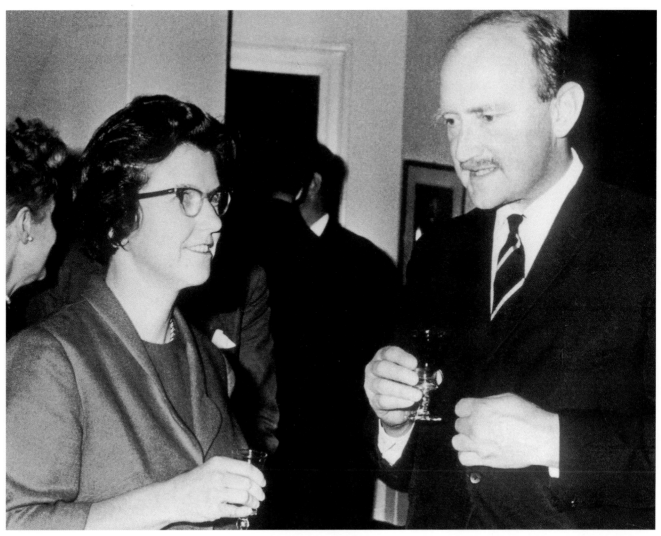

Hospital, and then joined Jere Mead, M.D., at the Harvard School of Public Health. Finally, by 1957—just five years after graduating from medical school and four years after her bout with tuberculosis—Avery was ready to take on the disease that had been stymieing the greatest minds in the field for decades. Following the thread that led from Pierre Simon Laplace's initial equation for the surface tension of curved surfaces through Neergaard's pioneering work and the more recent findings of Pattle, Clements, Mead, and others, Avery soon began to put the puzzle pieces together.

Her first clues came in the form of empirical findings. Unlike newborns who died from other causes, those who perished from hyaline membrane disease had no air in their lungs. Nor did they have pulmonary foam. Could it be, Avery wondered, that high surface tension in the lungs of infants lacking the foamy substance Clements had named "surfactant" might cause the alveoli to collapse?

As it turned out, it could. Experiments using a homemade surface-film balance (its design borrowed from Clements) allowed Avery to show

Mary Ellen Avery and Richard Pattle, two giants in the history of respiratory medicine, in 1965. A decade earlier, Pattle had studied the foamy fluid produced by human lungs, and found that it had remarkably low surface tension. Avery then built on Pattle and others' findings to identify the fluid as surfactant, which reduces surface tension in the lungs, allowing newborn lungs to expand just after birth.

Following spread: A world away from the old days: nurses work in a fully equipped neonatal unit. Advanced monitoring devices, mechanical ventilation, and such therapies as use of corticosteroids and surfactant replacement have helped reduce the annual death toll from Neonatal Respiratory Disease Syndrome to just over one thousand from the twenty thousand of half a century ago.

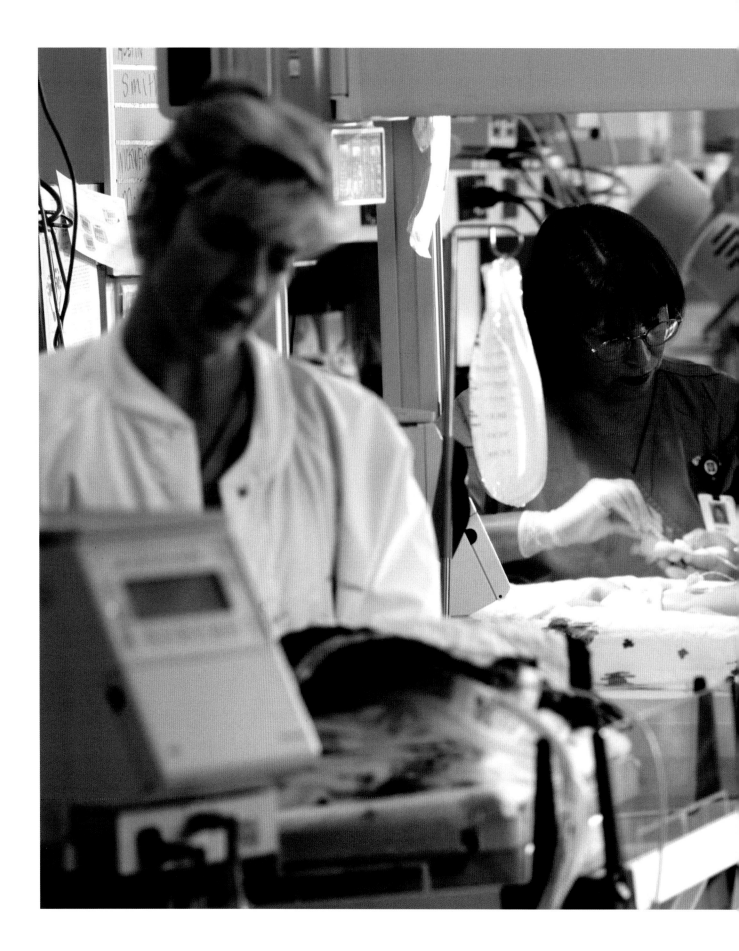

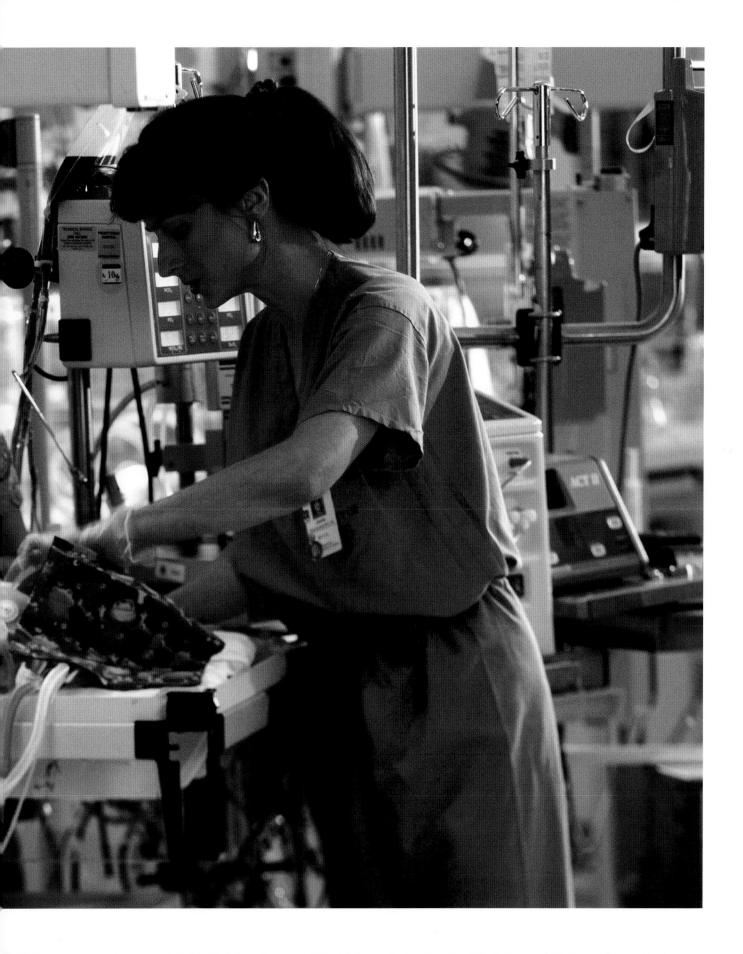

that while the surface tension of the foam in the lungs of adults, children, and infants who died from other causes decreased to 5–10 dynes/cm when compressed, the compressed lung extracts in the newborns who died from hyaline membrane disease—and therefore lacked the foam— maintained a surface tension of 20–30 dynes/cm. Avery also found that the lack of foam in certain newborns was associated with their prematurity. It appeared that these babies were born before their lungs had developed the ability to produce surfactant.

Avery's research, published in the *American Journal of Diseases of Children* in a 1959 article co-authored by Mead, and the resulting treatments have cut the death toll from NRDS to just over one thousand deaths per year of the forty thousand newborns who suffer from the syndrome.

Since production of surfactant (now known to be a mixture of lipids and proteins) begins at about thirty-four weeks of pregnancy, support of difficult pregnancies to minimize premature births remains the first weapon against NRDS. Amniocentesis allows obstetricians to determine if sufficient production of surfactant has begun. When premature delivery cannot be avoided, corticosteroids given to the mother cross the placenta and increase the fetal production of surfactant. Depending on the severity of the disease, oxygen at birth (delivered with a hood, using CPAP, or via intubation) can be used. Today, surfactant replacement therapy is known to dramatically improve or prevent many of the complications associated with NRDS. Surfactant, taken from calf or pig lungs or human amniotic fluid, or created synthetically, and instilled into the newborn's lungs through an endotracheal tube, helps the baby's lungs become more compliant, easier to ventilate, and require lower oxygen levels.

The story of surfactant and NRDS stands as a microcosm of the struggle to advance medical knowledge, both within the field of respiratory medicine and in medicine as a whole. The rapid advances of the 1950s show that the old barriers were finally falling, as researchers began to work together and build off each other's findings. Perhaps most important of all, the prominent presence of government sponsorship of basic research (through both the U.S. and British military, and in Mary Ellen Avery's NIH-sponsored training) foreshadows the increasingly important federal role in medical research. The combined efforts of the government— especially the military—and private research were also effective in attacking another seemingly incurable condition: Acute Respiratory Distress Syndrome (ARDS).

ARDS and the New Model of Medical Research

Just as World War I provided respiratory specialists with knowledge of the effects of poison gases on the lungs, and World War II produced

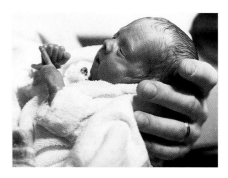

Adrienne Weber, the subject of Dr. Mary Ellen Avery's book *Born Early*. Born a mere one pound, nine ounces, Adrienne grew to be a healthy baby—largely due to Avery's pivotal research.

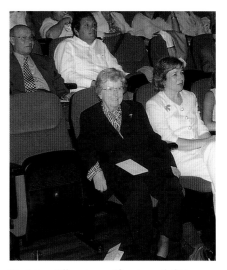

Dr. Mary Ellen Avery (front row, left) in 2002. Avery's initial, groundbreaking research into the role of surfactant in NRDS was sponsored by the National Institutes of Health—a harbinger of the critical role the NIH has since played in the battle against a host of diseases.

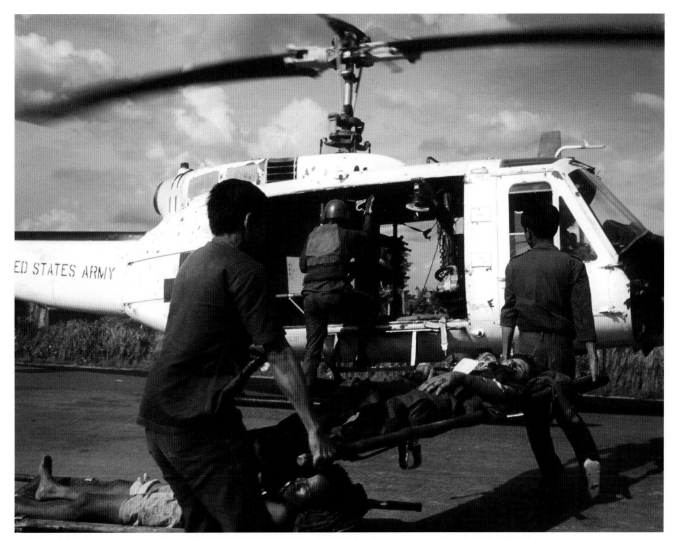

great technical advances in mechanical ventilation, the Vietnam War bequeathed its own appropriate memorial: the identification of a brutal, often-fatal condition in which injured soldiers who seemed to be recovering die suddenly from an inexplicable and devastating respiratory collapse.

Nearly forty years later, ARDS remains one of the most intractable enemies of respiratory medicine and critical care, affecting up to one hundred and fifty thousand people each year in the United States alone. Despite great advances in supporting patients with mechanical ventilation, the mortality rate from ARDS continues to hover at around 30 percent.

Long before the Vietnam War, physicians recognized that some trauma patients, apparently past the crisis stage, suddenly began suffering from acute respiratory distress, cyanosis, decreased lung compliance, and other rapidly developing and intractable symptoms. The condition, dubbed "shock lung" or "traumatic wet lung," was a central concern of the growing specialty of critical care medicine, and was an important reason behind the boom in intensive care units in the 1950s.

The Vietnam War will always be remembered by respiratory specialists as the conflict that led to deeper understanding of the catastrophic respiratory collapse that struck soldiers seemingly recovering from battlefield wounds. In 1967 a team of Colorado researchers identified the condition as Acute Respiratory Distress Syndrome (ARDS).

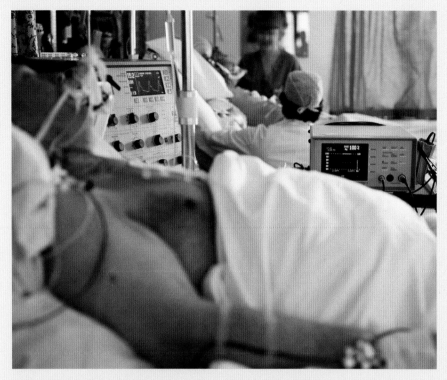

Wartime injuries often require immediate care, as many wounded soldiers will not survive being taken to a hospital miles away from the battlefield. This indisputable fact led to the development of the first medical and surgical units close to the front lines, in reality the first intensive-care units (ICUs).

The Development of ICUs and the Birth of Critical Care

One crucial development in the care of ARDS patients has been the development of respiratory intensive care units (ICUs)—indeed, of critical care as a specialty. And like many medical developments, there was a wartime link: the need to treat soldiers suffering from shock and trauma led to the creation of medical and surgical units close to the front lines. These were, in many respects, the first ICUs.

Hand in hand with the development of more advanced forms of mechanical ventilation came the arrival of ICUs in a hospital setting. Still, as of the late 1950s, barely a quarter of all large hospitals (those with more than three hundred beds) had an ICU. A decade later, the vast majority of hospitals had at least one. One pioneer in the field was Robert Rogers, who built the first respiratory intensive-care unit on the East Coast at the University of Pennsylvania. It served as a model for the units that soon sprouted up across the nation.

Permanent ICUs meant hospitals needed a permanent ICU staff—doctors, nurses, and technicians who had the latest training and information on how to care for their critically ill patients. The American Thoracic Society, with its many resources and extensive membership, was a natural link between all those involved with critical care.

The link is a necessary one—there are several varied occupations in critical care. Staff members include pulmonary/critical care-trained physicians who receive special education, training, and sub-specialty board certification specifically in critical care. But physicians are only part of the team required for critical care today.

Physicians work closely with critical-care nurses, who always receive highly specialized education and who are often certified in critical-care nursing as CCRNs. In many cases, it is the CCRN who has the closest contact with the patient and family, who functions most centrally as the patient's advocate, and who therefore becomes integral to the decision-making process of the entire critical-care team.

In addition, critical-care pharmacists and pharmacologists use their specialized training to monitor a patient's medications; respiratory therapists work with the team to monitor ventilators and other respiratory technology; and physical/occupational therapists, social workers, dieticians, and members of the clergy all play important roles as well.

Critical care is now a crucial part of the American Thoracic Society's mission. Since so much

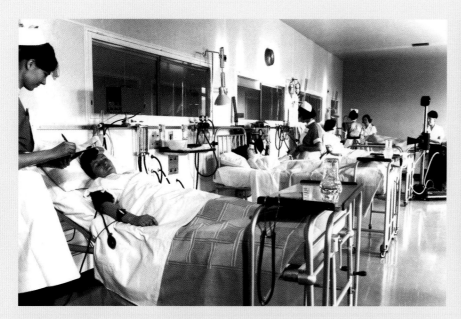

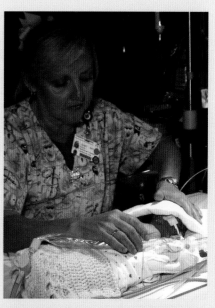

An early intensive-care ward in the Brompton Hospital, London, in 1969. As ICUs sprouted at more and more hospitals in the 1960s and 1970s, demand rose for physicians and nurses who were trained to treat ICU patients. New specialists—including physicians known as intensivists and critical-care nurses—soon came to fill the growing need.

A respiratory therapist with a premature baby. The hours after birth are critical to the survival of many premature babies and those with other health problems.

of the treatment of respiratory disease—from tuberculosis to NRDS, ARDS, and SARS— focuses on the care of critically ill patients, the Society has sought to elevate critical care to the prominence it deserves.

For example, the Assembly on Critical Care has the largest number of primary and secondary members of the Society's twelve assemblies. The Assembly on Critical Care reflects the international tenor that embodies the Society as a whole: one of its committees is an International Affairs Committee, and the chairs of this and other committees frequently include physicians from Europe and around the globe.

The mission of the Assembly on Critical Care is to prevent and fight diseases of the critically ill patient through research, education, patient care, and advocacy. The research component provides input to the Society's leadership for future directions in research and monitoring allocations of funding for critical care research. Similarly, goals in education focus on facilitating the interpretation and transfer of new knowledge to investigators, fellows in training, and practitioners; patient-care aims include continuously applying new knowledge to improve the care of critically ill patients; and the assembly's advocacy mission ensures increasing funding support of research.

Aside from the Assembly on Critical Care, the Society publishes frequent scientific statements and practice guidelines and sponsors and participates in international conferences on critical care. In addition, the Society takes an active part in: developing evidence-based critical care guidelines; advancing knowledge in hemodynamic monitoring; confronting critical-care billing issues; and helping establish a code for critical care ethics. All of these activities give truth to the American Thoracic Society's mission statement—that it is a "non-profit, international, professional and scientific society for respiratory *and* critical care medicine."

Still, the condition was neither understood nor studied intensively until the Vietnam War. At that time, the prevalence and toll of the syndrome began to become clear. It also acquired a new name: Da Nang Lung.

In 1967 a pair of Denver investigators, David Ashbaugh and Thomas Petty, finally provided a scientific description for what they ultimately called Acute Respiratory Distress Syndrome. "Previously, the condition had only been described in pathologic terms," Petty says. "Its characteristics were always determined on autopsy."

Ashbaugh and Petty were the first to attempt to treat the condition with mechanical ventilation. "We used an old ventilator, originally built during the polio epidemic in the mid-1950s," Petty recalls. "Fortunately, it had the capability for PEEP."

As a result of this breakthrough in treatment, Ashbaugh and Petty were able to study patients who had survived the acute crisis. The investigators began to identify the syndrome's precipitating factors, including sepsis, pneumonia, pulmonary aspiration, and burns. In addition, they began planning more refined treatment of the syndrome in an attempt to bring its high mortality rate—70 percent at the time—down.

But other specialists had trouble accepting that PEEP could be of benefit to patients with ARDS. When Ashbaugh and Petty submitted their initial findings to the *New England Journal of Medicine,* the response was rapid and unequivocal. "Our report came back very quickly with the scathing criticism that end-expiratory pressure had been proven to impair cardiac output by causing a reduction in venous return," Petty recalled in a 2001 article for the American Thoracic Society's *American Journal of Respiratory and Critical Care Medicine.*

Many even doubted that the syndrome, finally described by Ashbaugh and Petty in their groundbreaking 1967 *Lancet* article, existed. "For years after," Petty says, "there were still those who argued that it was not an entity at all." Today, fortunately, that debate seems to have been put to rest.

Still, even at the beginning, the Vietnam battlefield cases of ARDS were worrisome enough that in 1968—just a few months after it was first identified—the National Academy of Sciences summoned 125 military and civilian lung experts to an emergency conference to map out strategies to study and learn how to combat it. Meetings like this one, which warranted a mention in the *New York Times,* were still rare at the time.

But times were changing at last, as national—and even international—gatherings of experts became more and more commonplace, an important sign of the ongoing maturation of medicine as a whole. ARDS was a logical focus for the new model, bringing together a wide array of specialists seeking to contend with a condition that was hard to understand and even harder to treat.

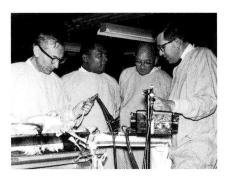

In 1967 Dr. David Ashbaugh (far right) and a team of University of Colorado investigators pulled together years of data and described Acute Respiratory Distress Syndrome (ARDS) for the first time. Their discovery led to a deeper understanding of ARDS, as well as improved treatment for the often-fatal syndrome.

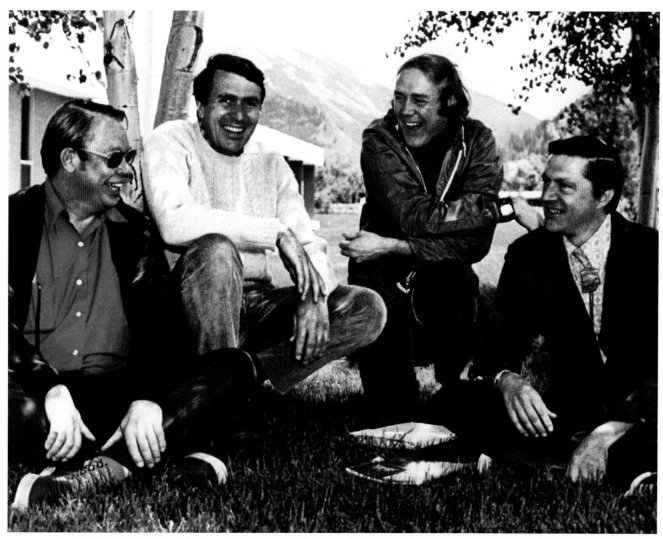

In recent years, researchers have made great strides in understanding the pathophysiology and clinical manifestations of ARDS. They've also succeeded in reducing the mortality rate to about 30 percent—still frighteningly high, but far lower than it was when the syndrome was first identified.

The ARDS Network (ARDS Net) is an ambitious collaborative effort created by the NHLBI to seek out new, more effective ways to treat ARDS—and perhaps even find a cure. Begun in 1994, it includes nineteen clinical centers (comprised of forty-four hospitals) that coordinate studies, develop protocols, and undertake multicenter studies to test the effectiveness of drugs such as ketoconazole and ventilation techniques to lower the mortality rate of this syndrome.

For ARDS patients, the close care and supervision they receive from critical-care specialists in respiratory ICUs frequently means the difference between life and death. More than thirty-five years after Ashbaugh and Petty used an old respirator to provide support to their patients, PEEP remains a mainstay of therapy.

Before researchers (from left to right) William Thurlbeck, David Ashbaugh, Len Hudson, and Thomas Petty at the University of Colorado set to work, ARDS had been identified only by pathologic examination after death of the patient. As well as identifying it in living patients, Petty and the group were also the first to use mechanical ventilation to prolong patients' lives.

Other ventilation choices in ARDS have been refined over the years. Originally, mechanical ventilation with higher-than-normal tidal volumes was used to ventilate ARDS patients, following the theory that the patients' "stiff lungs" (due to edema) required it. Not until trials sponsored by ARDS Net showed that high tidal volumes can exacerbate lung injury did current treatments with lower tidal volumes come into widespread use.

A variety of pharmacologic treatments have also been attempted. They include inhaled nitric oxide, corticosteroids, and instillation of pulmonary surfactant into the lungs. As of yet, however, none of these therapies has shown any significant clinical benefit. Future progress, says Petty, depends on an imaginative, dogma-challenging approach, one that addresses the basic biological processes of ARDS.

For the physician, the respiratory therapist, and the public alike, battling such an intractable syndrome provides ongoing proof of the need for a united effort to seek new insights not only into ARDS, but also into a myriad of other syndromes and diseases. Each group can play to its own strength: American Thoracic Society members undertake research into the basic science, symptoms, and treatment of ARDS. Meanwhile, other public-health organizations can sponsor campaigns to increase knowledge and reduce fear about the syndrome, and the informed public can advocate for increased governmental funding and more aggressive research.

This kind of "perfect storm" approach to studying, treating, and publicizing a disease or syndrome would have seemed like a fantasy a generation ago. In the age of emerging viruses such as AIDS and SARS, however, with tuberculosis resurgent, and ARDS still claiming an enormous toll, it is a method that will clearly play a crucial role in the ongoing—and ever-evolving—battle against respiratory disease.

Sleep and the Lungs

The unified approach to confronting respiratory conditions has never been employed more aggressively than in sleep medicine, a specialty that only recently was recognized, but which now is a necessary addition to the list of new-millennium respiratory challenges.

In the eighth century B.C., the Greek poet Hesiod called sleep "the brother of death." In 1834 the Scottish physician Robert MacNish went into more detail, writing, "Sleep is the intermediate state between wakefulness and death: wakefulness is regarded as the active state of all animal and intellectual functions and death as that of their total suspension."

But this sort of empirical, poetic finding was all that philosophers and physicians alike had to work with for centuries. There was no way

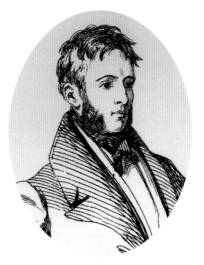

Both a surgeon and popular writer, Robert MacNish's treatise, "Philosophy of Sleep," was widely read all over Europe and America. However, as little was known about sleep at the time, the work was more metaphysical than scientific.

to actually try to figure out why we slept, or what went on when we did. Of course, this didn't stop the promulgation of a variety of "scientific" theories to explain what we didn't know. Sleep, some said, was due to congestion of pressure of blood in the brain. No, argued others; it took place to drain away the toxic substances (including cholesterol and carbon dioxide) that accumulated during wakeful hours.

In the nineteenth century, a handful of scientists began to look deeper. Researchers began to identify the link between the brain and sleep by noting that animal subjects entered a permanent state of "sleepiness" when certain portions of the brain were removed. Others, noting the rhythmic nature of sleep and wakefulness, began to pinpoint other bodily changes associated with the chronobiology of sleep. Certain sleep disorders, including insomnia, "Pickwickian Syndrome," and narcolepsy, were identified.

Then, in the late 1920s, a German psychiatrist named Hans Berger used primitive string galvanometers to chart the electrical brain signals of humans during wakefulness and sleep. Berger wasn't the first to measure the brain's electrical activity, but he was the first to undertake careful, repeatable readings on the subject. In doing so, he became the first to employ the electroencephalogram (EEG).

Reporting on his first findings in 1929, Berger wrote: "We see in the electroencephalogram a concomitant phenomenon of the continuous nerve processes which take place in the brain, exactly as the electrocardiogram represents a concomitant phenomenon of the contractions of the individual segments of the heart." Within two years, Berger had taken more than a thousand readings from seventy-six subjects; named alpha and beta waves; found that epileptic patients had large-amplitude waves; and noted that alpha waves diminished during sleep, general anesthesia, and cocaine use.

The medical community roundly ignored Berger's initial findings. Since conventional wisdom held that brain-wave recordings were impossible to interpret, why should anyone listen to a quiet German psychiatrist who claimed otherwise? Only when Berger's findings were replicated in England in the 1930s did he receive the attention he deserved and did the science of sleep medicine evolve further.

Berger never got to see his discoveries put to further use. Persecuted by the Nazis, who forced him to resign his university position and prohibited him from accepting international awards, he committed suicide in 1941. But others carried on his work (in fits and starts), gradually using EEGs and other methods to define various stages of sleep, most importantly REM sleep, which was first identified in 1957 by Nathaniel Kleitman and Eugene Aserinsky at the University of Chicago.

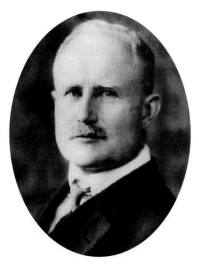

Too often, crucial advances in medicine must fight through a barrage of skepticism before they become accepted practice. For example, deep-rooted beliefs that brain-waves were impossible to interpret made experts ignore the contrary findings of the German psychiatrist Hans Berger, the first to use an electroencephalogram (EEG).

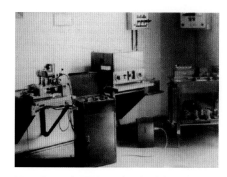

Hans Berger's EEG, with which he identified and named alpha and beta brainwaves and discovered that alpha waves diminish during sleep. Once accepted, Berger's 1929 findings opened the door to a deeper understanding of sleep—as well as treatment for sleep disorders.

By the 1960s, several sleep research laboratories had opened in the United States and Europe. These, however, were seen as research tools with little or no clinical application. The concept that disorders of sleep might contribute to serious medical conditions was still not widely accepted. Despite several forays in that direction, it took many more years—until the 1980s—before sleep disorders began to be considered as part of the panoply of serious medical conditions.

John Remmers, M.D., was the first person to explain why the breathing passage closes in sleep apnea, and this explanation provides a textbook example of the roadblocks faced by those who chose to specialize in sleep medicine just thirty years ago. The condition had already been named Pickwickian Syndrome, after a character in a Dickens' novel, and was characterized by obesity, excessive daytime sleepiness, shortness of breath, heart failure, and other symptoms. The syndrome had been blamed on "carbon dioxide narcosis," or on obesity's compromising of respiratory muscles, but these were, in truth, just guesses.

It is now known that obstructive sleep apnea has many respiratory causes and effects. However, it has become much more prevalent outside the pulmonary community for many reasons. Obstructive sleep apnea increases with age and obesity, two conditions affecting more and more Americans. Additionally, it has major public health repercussions due to increased daytime somnolence (drowsiness), causing car accidents. Obstructive sleep apnea may also cause systemic hypertension, which affects thousands of people with cardiovascular diseases. It is also significant in other, more common diseases such as heart failure, asthma, and chronic obstructive pulmonary disease (COPD). In spite of all these concerns, little was known about the disease until Remmers investigated further.

In 1974, while working at the University of Texas Medical Branch in Galveston, Remmers sought to determine the real cause of the condition. "I used an early oximeter to measure blood oxygen, and a cardiac transducer to measure pressures in the esophagus," Remmers recalls. "They showed that supraglottic pressure and esophageal pressure was transmitted through the larynx to the pharynx. I'd spent five years studying the larynx, and had hoped to find an obstruction there—but it was clear that the obstruction was of pharyngeal origin."

Remmers then teamed up with Eberhardt K. Sauerland, M.D., a colleague in Galveston. "It was such pure luck," Remmers says. "He'd studied the activity of the genioglossus muscle, and had discovered that it had a respiratory function. Together, we were able to detail the roles of pharyngeal collapse and the genioglossus in causing what is now known as obstructive sleep apnea."

As so often happens, the initial description of the condition led to an explosion of research into its causes, sequelae, and treatments.

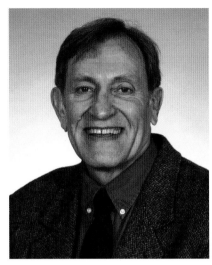

Though he expected to find that an obstruction in the larynx caused obstructive sleep apnea, Dr. John Remmers of the University of Texas Medical Branch found that the condition actually originated in the pharynx.

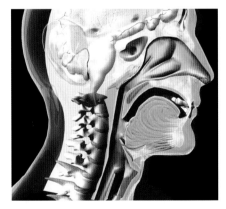

The human oral and nasal cavity. Dr. John Remmers and others have demonstrated an intricate series of interactions involving the larynx, pharynx, tongue, and brain that together lie at the heart of obstructive sleep apnea.

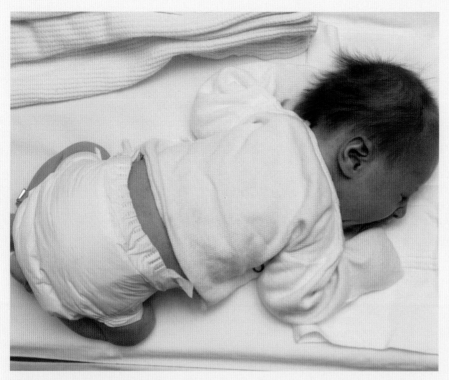

Sudden infant death syndrome (SIDS) continues to be one of the most intensively studied, yet least-understood conditions in sleep medicine. Despite many advances in understanding the causes of the syndrome, SIDS remains the leading cause of death in young infants.

Sudden Infant Death Syndrome

Of all the disorders studied and treated by experts in sleep medicine, by far the most baffling and heartbreaking remains sudden infant death syndrome, more commonly known as SIDS. Despite years of research and a plethora of studies, its exact cause—why one baby dies suddenly and quietly during sleep, while another does not—remains a mystery. Even its diagnosis is one of exclusion, settled upon when an autopsy has proven that accidents, abuse, and previously undiagnosed conditions are not to blame.

However, the intense focus on SIDS had produced a variety of life-saving findings. In particular, researchers have identified a set of important risk factors that increase the chances that a baby will die of SIDS. While no one risk factor is thought to be sufficient to cause SIDS, a combination of factors may contribute to an infant's death.

Among the risk factors for SIDS are:
• Ethnicity: African-American infants are two times more likely to die of SIDS than are Caucasian infants, while Native Americans

are three times as likely
• Smoking, drinking, and drug use during pregnancy
• Prematurity and/or low birth weight
• Smoke exposure
• Sleeping on the stomach during the first months of life

This last factor appears to be the most crucial risk factor yet determined. Up until about a decade ago, the accepted sleep position for infants was on the stomach to minimize the chance of babies choking on vomitus.

But studies in the 1980s began to show a higher incidence of SIDS in babies who slept on their stomachs than in those who slept on their backs or sides. Hypotheses for why this might be so include pressure on the child's jaw which interfered with breathing; the infant's "rebreathing" stale, exhaled air (especially while sleeping on a soft mattress or with bedding close to the face); or a defect in the arcuate nucleus, an area of the brain that normally alerts infants to wake and cry when the brain is not getting enough oxygen.

In 1992 the American Academy of Pediatrics recommended that infants younger than one year be placed on their backs to sleep. Intensive publicity campaigns by the Academy and other organizations have helped spread the word, and SIDS rates dropped by more than 40 percent from 1992 to 1997.

Even with all these advances, SIDS remains the leading cause of death in young infants, but scientists remain committed to eradicating this mysterious syndrome.

In 1981, an Australian physician named Colin Sullivan invented nasal coninuous positive airway pressure (CPAP), originally as a technique for studying sleep apnea. It quickly became apparent that it was an effective treatment for the condition—one that is still in widespread use today.

As the critical importance of sleep disorders began to be realized, the NIH established the National Center on Sleep Disorders Research (NCSDR) within the NHLBI. The NCSDR's first research plan, released in 1996, called for the center "to improve the health, safety, and productivity of Americans by promoting basic, clinical, and applied research on sleep and sleep disorders." It focused on a variety of different disorders, including what is now called Sleep-Disordered Breathing (SDB), an umbrella term describing obstructive and central sleep apnea and other conditions such as Cheyne-Stokes respiration.

The Sleep Heart Health Study, an ongoing, critically important long-term study undertaken under the auspices of the NHLBI, seeks to test a series of hypotheses about the effects of SDB on the heart. The study, begun in 1995 and including about sixty-four hundred individuals studied at seven research centers, will quantify the extent to which SDB is associated with coronary heart disease events, stroke, increased blood pressure, all-around mortality, and a variety of other conditions.

Under the NIH's broad mandate, and a second plan released in 2003, due attention was finally paid to sleep-disorder research and treatment. At last, the concept that what happens during sleep has a critical impact on health became a bedrock principle of modern medicine.

The recent intensive focus on sleep disorders has already yielded great benefits. Studies of the respiratory components of sudden infant death syndrome (SIDS) have dramatically changed the recommendations for infant sleep position, saving thousands of lives. And research into such pediatric disorders as Congenital Central Hypoventilation Syndrome and Rett Syndrome—a neurobiological disease characterized in part by hyperventilation and apnea while awake—has led to a far greater understanding of autonomic regulation and respiratory control.

In many ways, the recent advances in understanding, identification, and treatment of sleep disorders mirror those of earlier challenges ranging from tuberculosis to NRDS. In each case, early findings were hindered by long-held misconceptions, international barriers to cooperation, and other missteps. Only when these prejudices were overcome, as the American Thoracic Society had long advocated, did new eras of collegiality begin—eras that led to rapid advances in basic research, improvements in public health and education, and, in many cases, treatments and cures that had long seemed beyond reach.

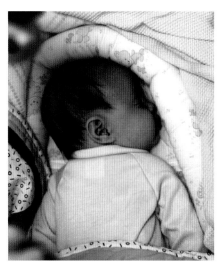

A critically important way to reduce the number of deaths from SIDS involves sleep position. In the 1990s, sleep experts realized that previous recommendations—that infants be placed on their stomachs—were wrong. Babies must be placed on their backs and away from soft cushions, saggy mattresses, or heavy blankets that can interfere with breathing.

Opposite: Sleep medicine has come a long way since Hans Berger's first primitive EEG machine. Today, the disipline relies on complex scanning and monitoring devices that provide a detailed view into the workings of the lungs and central nervous system during sleep, as shown here at the McGill University Health Center Laboratory in Montreal, Quebec.

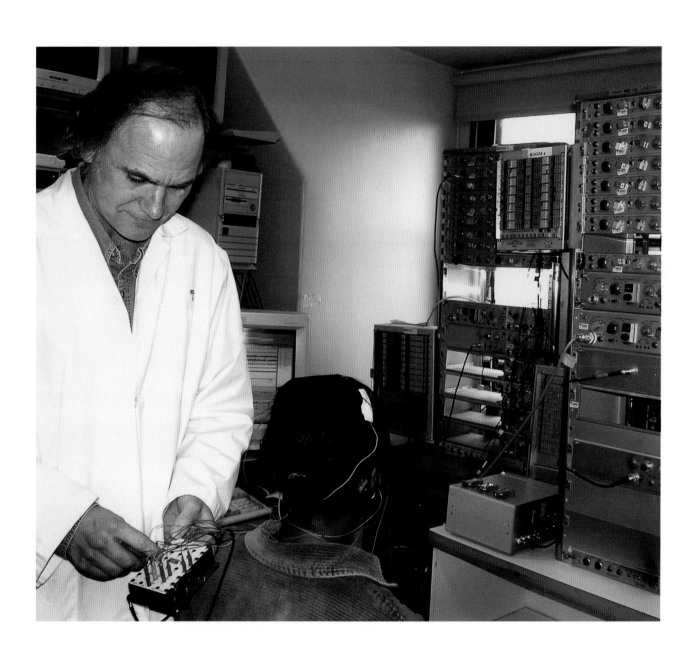

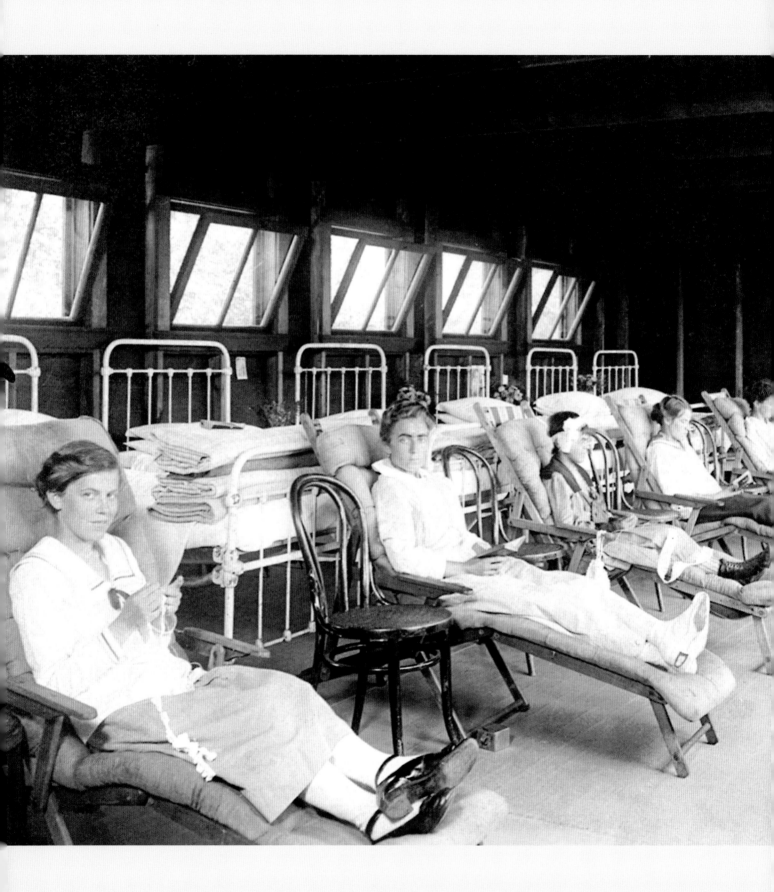

CHAPTER THREE

1905–2005

A Century of Progress:
Pivotal Moments in Respiratory Health

Respiratory health has made monumental leaps in the last century. Despite facing incredibly powerful diseases, healthcare professionals have helped to prevent lung disease, promote lung health, and enhance patient care worldwide. These achievements, however, have not come easily. As Julius Comroe writes in *Retrospectroscope: Insights into Medical Discovery*, there is no "simple or royal road to success in medical discovery . . . . [Scientists] are human, take wrong turns, travel tortuous paths, and sometimes arrive because of someone else's speculation or unrelated observation, or by chance (*plus* sagacity)."

The paths in science and medicine may not be easy, but they are all crucial to the development of modern respiratory health. The following timeline features the respiratory programs, inventions, legislative action, and pivotal moments that have occurred over the last hundred years. Working with scientists and healthcare professionals, the American Thoracic Society has supported research and created an international forum, translating these developments into education, patient care, and advocacy programs. But this timeline is more than just a chronicle of past achievements—the dedication and hope involved reveal a bright future for the worldwide treatment of respiratory health.

Opposite: The past century has seen an almost incomprehensible leap in our ability to treat and prevent respiratory diseases that once took an enormous toll. Within a single generation, for example, tuberculosis went from killing thousands each year—and condemning others to long stays in sanatoriums—to being a disease that can be cured through a carefully followed drug regimen.

1905
American Sanatorium Association is founded as part of the ALA. At this time, dues were one dollar per year.

ATS

APRIL 15, 1912
The world's largest passenger ship, the Titanic, sinks four hours after hitting an iceberg.

1905

Robert Koch, who in 1882 discovered *Mycobacterium tuberculosis*, the bacillus that causes tuberculosis, receives the Nobel Prize for Physiology or Medicine for the discovery that led to the first effective treatments for the disease.

1907

Clemens von Pirquet and Charles Mantoux introduce safe, effective skin tests for tuberculosis, using **tuberculin**. For the first time, the disease can be positively diagnosed in infants and excluded in adults.

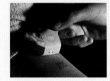

1909

Willy Meyer installs his **"Universal Negative Pressure Chamber"** for pulmonary surgery in the Rockefeller Institute in New York City. One thousand cubic feet in volume, it is able to contain 17 people, including patient, surgeon, assistants, an engineer, and two anesthetists.

1911

Artificial pneumothorax, first reported in 1894 in Europe, is performed successfully on a patient with tuberculosis in the United States. It ushers in an era of lung collapse therapy that will soon include plombage, pneumoperitoneum, and phrenic nerve collapse.

1912

The Marine Hospital Service, parent organization

to the National Institutes of Health and originally created to contend with the often intractable diseases brought back by sailors, is renamed the **United States Public Health Service**. Its charter is expanded to include research into such diseases as tuberculosis, malaria, and leprosy.

1913

The **Kansas City Gas Company**, specializing in oxygen and nitrous oxide compressed gases, is formed. Later, it will evolve into a producer of ventilator systems, oxygen therapy, and other respiratory products.

JANUARY 19, 1915
Gandhi returns to India to begin his non-violent protest against British rule which would lead to India's emancipation.

1915

Edward Livingston Trudeau, a towering figure in the struggle against tuberculosis and the founder of the first sanatorium in North America, dies of complications from his own tuberculosis.

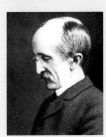

1920

The National Association for the Study and Prevention of Tuberculosis (later the **American Lung Association**) embarks on an ambitious research program, initially focusing on scientific improvements in X-rays and the tuberculin test. More than six decades later, in the 1980s, the ALA undertakes a significant revision of the program. It will establish the "career ladder" program, which awards funding to individuals in academic settings working in lung research.

1922

Jean Sicard and Jacques Forestier first describe **bronchography**, which

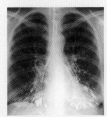

becomes widely used to diagnose bronchiectasis and to plot the involved segments for surgery. Today, bronchography has mostly been abandoned for less invasive imaging techniques.

1928

Following the observations and experiments of Pasteur, Lister, Joubert, and others, Alexander Fleming discovers **penicillin**. The first human test comes in 1941—and within a few years, penicillin and many other antibiotics will revolutionize medical treatment for pneumonia and many other diseases.

1929

Philip Drinker and Louis Agassiz Shaw announce the invention of the **iron lung**, which mimics natural breathing patterns in patients with chest paralysis. In an era of nearly annual polio epidemics, the iron lung serves as a lifesaver for thousands of patients with the disease.

Hans Berger, an Austrian psychiatrist, publishes the results of 73 recordings of brain electrical activity. These and subsequent readings, the first **EEGs**, find that alpha waves diminish during sleep and general anesthesia and that epilepsy, Alzheimer's disease, and multiple sclerosis all also alter EEG readings.

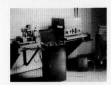

OCTOBER 24, 1945
The United Nations is formed immediately after World War II to maintain peace and solve humanitarian problems.

1929

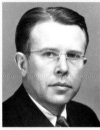

Ernest O. Lawrence invents the **cyclotron** at the University of California's Radiation Laboratory in Berkeley, California. The cyclotron will soon produce the first medically useful radionuclides, which are indispensable tools for investigations of normal and abnormal lungs. In 1939 Lawrence will receive the Nobel Prize in Physics for his invention.

1934

Two decades after Robert Koch's development of tuberculin, a failed treatment for tuberculosis, Florence Siebert prepares **purified protein derivative (PPD)** from tuberculin. PPD soon becomes an important research tool—as well as the basis for a widely used, extremely accurate skin test for latent tuberculosis infection.

1940s

Like many other inventors, technical training officer Forrest Bird helps design **oxygen masks** that enable World War II pilots to fly at higher altitudes than ever before. After the war ends, Bird uses his hard-won expertise to produce the first universal medical respirator.

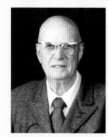

1944

Selman Waksman and others first test **streptomycin** in a human subject suffering from tuberculosis. Within a decade, an array of

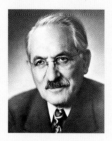

other antibiotics—including isoniazid, para-aminosalicylic acid, and pyrazinamide—are being used, alone and in combination, to treat tuberculosis.

1945

The first **vaccine against influenza** becomes available in the United States, helping control a disease that had killed as many as 40 million people worldwide in a single epidemic (1918–19). Today, nasal "live" vaccines have joined the traditional killed vaccines as scientists continue to battle other roadblocks—vulnerable individuals who fail to take the vaccine as well as vaccine availability.

Ernest Huant, a physician who regularly uses nicotinamide to reduce nausea and vomiting in patients undergoing radiation therapy, observes clearing of densities in chest films of patients with tuberculosis. Huant brings his findings to the attention of tuberculosis specialists, who soon isolate **isoniazid**, a nicotinamide derivative that becomes one of the most powerful weapons against tuberculosis.

1946

The **Communicable Disease Center (CDC)** opens in Atlanta with the mission of combating malaria, typhus, and other diseases still prevalent in southern states. In the following years, the CDC—eventually named the Centers for Disease Control—expands its mission, playing a crucial role in the identification of Legionnaire's disease, hantavirus, Ebola, and other diseases.

1947

Wallace Fenn, Hermann Rahn, Arthur Otis, and Leigh Chadwick publish their groundbreaking work on **pulmonary gas exchange**: a graphical analysis that relates an astonishing six variables: PO_2, PCO_2, respiratory exchange ratio, arterial oxygen saturation, alveolar ventilation, and altitude.

Physicians, nurses, and other "oxygen orderlies" meet at the University of Chicago to form the **Inhalational Therapy Association**. Early members are expected to be able to do acute-care hospital tasks ranging from repairing equipment to formulating a budget.

1948

J. W. Coltman of Westinghouse introduces an image intensifier that allows a dramatic gain in **brightness during fluoroscopy**. For the first time, television display becomes possible, as does recording of images in motion.

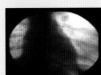

1950

Cortisone, a steroid originally extracted from the human adrenal gland in 1936, is first used as a treatment for asthma. By the 1970s, a refined, inhalable corticosteroid called beclomethasone will be widely used in aerosol inhalers to prevent acute asthma attacks. Today, five inhaled corticosteroids are used for asthma maintenance therapy in the United States.

1953

Gordon Brownell at MIT constructs the first detector

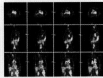

device to exploit **positron annihilation** as an imaging tool. This device is the first precursor of Positron Emission Tomography (PET) scanners.

JANUARY 8, 1954
*Elvis pays Sun
Studios in Memphis,
Tennessee, four
dollars to record his
first two songs.*

1953

Leland Clark
develops a platinum
electrode for **direct
measurement of
PO$_2$** which reflects
the level of oxygen
in the blood.

1954

The **sanatorium
movement** reaches
its peak, with more
than 100,000 beds
set aside for tuber-
culosis in the United
States alone. But the
fate of sanatoria has
already been set, and
within a decade, the
widespread use of
effective antibiotics
will see the closing
of nearly every
sanatorium in
the nation.

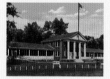

1955

Polio, an epidemic
disease that struck
over 20,000 individ-
uals (mostly chil-
dren) each year in
the United States,
is finally brought
under control by
Jonas Salk's killed-
virus vaccine. Seven
years later, Albert
Sabin unveils a
significant advance:
an oral "live"
vaccine, which pro-
vides both intestinal
and bodily immu-
nity while requiring
no booster shot.

DeFrancis and
others demonstrate
that **needle biopsy
of the pleura**,
performed under
local anesthetic,
allows for quick
diagnosis of tubercu-
losis, cancer, and
other diseases in
patients who have
been suffering from
persistent pleural
effusion.

1956

DuBois, Botelho,
and Comroe (below)
use a **body plethys-
mograph** to meas-

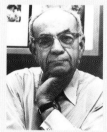

ure airway resistance
in normal individu-
als and those with
respiratory disease.
This is one of
several pulmonary
function tests
performed routinely
to diagnose and
stage lung disease.

Werner Forssmann,
Andre Cournand,
and Dickinson
Richards share the
Nobel Prize in
physiology and
medicine for their
contributions to the
advancement of
**right-heart
catheterization**.
Their work leads to
the development in
the early 1970s of
the balloon-tipped
Swan-Ganz catheter.
The catheter, like
the 2000 model
here, is still the most
widely used method
for assessing heart
function and meas-
uring pulmonary
hemodynamics.

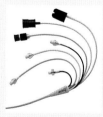

1957

Charles Sidney Burwell recognizes **obstructive sleep apnea syndrome**, which he names "Pickwickian Syndrome" after a character in Dickens's *The Pickwick Papers*. Burwell's description leads to an explosion of research about and new treatments for the syndrome.

1959

Richard Riley, an investigator at Johns Hopkins University, demonstrates that **tuberculosis can be spread via droplet nuclei**, minuscule droplets containing no more than three *M. tuberculosis* bacilli. Transmitted by talking, coughing, or sneezing, droplet nuclei are so small that they can remain airborne for extended periods of time.

Mary Ellen Avery and Jere Mead determine that some

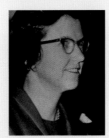

newborn babies' lungs do not produce surfactant, a critically important substance that enables neonates to breathe by reducing surface tension in the lining of the lungs. What has long been called **"hyaline membrane disease"** is soon more commonly called neonatal respiratory distress syndrome, or NRDS.

The Arden House Conference of leading tuberculosis experts recommends aggressive use of chemotherapy to fully eradicate the disease in the United States.

1960s

Short-acting bronchodilators known as **beta-agonists** are established as an effective rescue medication for patients with asthma. Early versions have significant side-effects, but by 1982, inhaled beta-agonists become the frontline treatment of acute asthma attacks. The introduction of inhaled long-acting beta-agonists in 1993 add yet another effective weapon against asthma.

1960

In the late 1950s, James Elam and Peter Safar refine and update mouth-to-mouth ventilation, a resuscitation technique known from Biblical times but long neglected. In 1960 Jude, Kouwenhoven, and Knickerbocker discover the benefits of chest compression to achieve artificial circulation. The two procedures are soon combined to form **modern-day cardiopulmonary resuscitation,** or CPR.

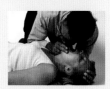

1960

Physician and avid climber Charles Houston first identifies **high-altitude pulmonary edema (HAPE)** as a life-threatening clinical syndrome featuring leakage of proteins into the lungs, possibly due to increased intracapillary pressure forcing basement membrane cells apart. Prior to the work of Houston and others, pulmonary deaths at altitude were always attributed to acute cardiac failure or pneumonia.

Allison and others perform the first successful **pulmonary thromboendarterectomy** in a patient with thromboembolic disease, though in

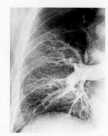

this first case they remove only fresh clots. Today, the procedure has become the definitive treatment for chronic thromboembolism.

1961

The American Thoracic Society releases a **statement on smoking and health**, describing an alarming rise in deaths from lung cancer due to cigarette smoking and stating smoking's likely role in contributing to such other respiratory diseases as emphysema and chronic bronchitis.

The American Thoracic Society and the National Tuberculosis Association urge the United States Public Health Service to wage war on respiratory diseases resulting from **air pollution**— becoming among the first health organizations to make air pollution a health issue.

1963

Sten Ericksson discovers that a deficiency in the blood of a protein called **alpha-1 antitrypsin**, which normally serves to protect the lungs from the effects of powerful enzymes known as elastases, is an important cause of emphysema. This finding will lead to the development of alpha-1 antitrypsin replacement therapy, one of the emphysema treatments in use today.

1964

Shigeto Ikeda of the National Cancer Institute, Tokyo, develops the first **flexible fiberoptic bronchoscope**. Far less unwieldy than previous rigid models, the device allows for evaluation and imaging of smaller airways of the lung, and is also the leading tool for diagnosis of bronchogenic carcinoma.

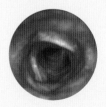

DECEMBER 3, 1967
Christiaan Barnard performs the first heart transplant in Cape Town, South Africa.

JULY 20, 1969
Apollo 11, manned by Neil Armstrong, Michael Collins, and Edwin Aldrin Jr., lands on the moon.

1967   1968   1969

U.S. surgeon general Luther Terry, working with the

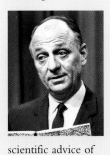

scientific advice of American Thoracic Society experts and others, releases the ground-breaking *Report on Smoking and Health*. For the first time, a federal agency lays out the indisputable evidence that smoking contributes to lung cancer, emphysema, chronic bronchitis, coronary heart disease, and other diseases.

Tom Petty and others at the University of Colorado Health Science Center in Denver identify a common outcome of patients with shock, trauma, massive infections, and other conditions resulting in acute respiratory distress.

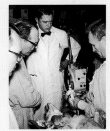

The syndrome, known since World War I, most frequently seen in battlefield injuries, and known during the Vietnam era as "Da Nang Lung," is initially named *Adult Respiratory Distress Syndrome (ARDS)*.

After years of effort, two teams of researchers, the Ishizaka Group in Denver, Colorado, and Bennich and Johensson from Sweden, identify the structure and antigenicity of a new immunoglobulin, which they name *IgE*. This discovery opens the door to a deeper understanding of the mechanisms of allergies and other hypersensitivity reactions, as well as allowing the development of improved diagnoses and treatment.

Researchers define *sudden infant death syndrome*

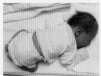

(SIDS) as "the sudden death of any infant or young child, which is unexpected by history, and in which a thorough postmortem examination fails to demonstrate an adequate cause for death."

The *National Heart Institute (NHI)* reorganizes to establish five program branches, including one on pulmonary disease. As a result of the reorganization, the institute is renamed the National Heart and Lung Institute (NHLI), on its way to its current name, the National Heart, Lung, and Blood Institute (NHLBI).

The *Federal Coal Mine and Safety Act* becomes law, seeking to reduce the amount of coal dust allowed in mines. The law aims to prevent cases of coal workers' pneumoconiosis (CWP), more commonly known as black lung disease, long known to be caused by long-term exposure to coal dust.

FEBRUARY 21, 1972
U.S. president Richard Nixon begins an eight-day visit to Communist China and meets with Mao Zedong.

1970s

The establishment of **intensive care units** in hospitals as specialized environments for treating critical illnesses becomes more widespread throughout the country.

1970

Congress passes—and President Nixon signs—the **Clean Air Act**, landmark legislation imposing federal regulations on a host of airborne pollutants. The Act results from years of scientific research and lobbying by the American Thoracic Society, American Lung Association, and other organizations.

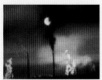

The **Occupational Health and Safety Act** becomes law, ushering in a new era in public efforts to protect workers from job-related injuries.

1971

The **National Institute for Occupational Safety and Health (NIOSH)** is established. The institute is responsible for conducting research and making recommendations for the prevention of work-related illnesses and injuries including those of the lung.

1972

Computed tomography (CT) is simultaneously and

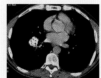

independently invented by Godfrey Hounsfield and Allan Cormack, and the men share the 1979 Nobel Prize for the invention. Today, more than 30,000 hospitals and health centers worldwide utilize CT technology.

1975

The **Parker B. Francis Fellowship** program is established. Receiving more than $30 million in contributions from the Francis Families Foundation, the program continues to sponsor young investigators studying lung biology, pulmonary disease, and anesthesiology.

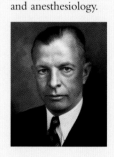

JULY 4, 1976
The United States celebrates its bicentennial.

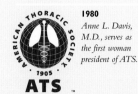

1980
Anne L. Davis, M.D., serves as the first woman president of ATS.

ATS

1976

Extracorporeal membrane oxygenation (ECMO) is introduced to provide lung support in neonates with persistent pulmonary hypertension of the newborn. Utilizing a heart-lung machine, ECMO gives the newborn's own lungs time to heal and recover.

1978

Robert Furchgott describes "endothelium-derived

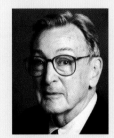

relaxing factor," an endogenous vasodilator now known as **nitric oxide**, for which he later receives the Nobel Prize. Today, nitric oxide is recognized to play a vital role in vascular and neuronal physiology, and is the focus of major research in lung, brain, and many other cellular functions.

The **Mine Safety and Health Administration (MSHA)** is created within the Labor Department, following passage of the Federal Mine Safety and Health Act of 1977. Immediately, MSHA's Coal Mine Safety and Health division begins conducting over 50,000 inspections and accident investigations each year, and writing 120,000 citations annually.

1980s

The invention of the power slip ring allows CT scanners to rotate continuously at a steady speed, enabling them to undertake "spiral" scanning. **Spiral CT scanners** can now image the lungs or other anatomic regions in a single 20–30 second breath hold, acquiring significant data with the patient's anatomy in a single position. Spiral CT has opened new avenues of investigation into lung structure and function.

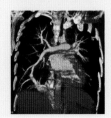

A team of researchers led by A. Charles Bryan of the Hospital for Sick Children, Toronto, devises a means of **high-frequency ventilation** (also known as high-frequency oscillation) that appears to provide significant benefits in infants suffering from neonatal respiratory distress syndrome (NRDS).

1980

The British **nocturnal oxygen therapy trial** reveals that long-term domiciliary oxygen therapy for at least 15 hours a day significantly improves survival over nocturnal therapy in patients with severe hypoxemic chronic obstructive pulmonary disease (COPD). A second long-term, multicenter trial in the United States and Canada, undertaken under the auspices of the National Heart, Lung, and Blood Institute (NHLBI) reaches similar conclusions.

1980

Colin Sullivan uses a two-stage vacuum-cleaner motor, individually molded masks, and the inside of a bicycle helmet to create the first device to deliver **continuous positive airway pressure (CPAP)**

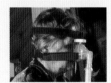

to patients with obstructive sleep apnea. Once perfected, the device—which delivers air to the airway through a specially designed mask at a high enough pressure to prevent apneas—becomes the therapeutic tool of choice for patients with this condition.

1981

The Centers for Disease Control report surprising recent incidence of cytomegalovirus, *Pneumocystis carinii* pneumonia, Kaposi sarcoma, and high death rates in gay men treated at hospitals nationwide. What is first called Gay-Related Immunodeficiency Disease will soon become known as **Acquired Immune Deficiency Syndrome**, or **AIDS**.

1982

Selective beta-2 agonists are approved for use in patients with asthma. These quickly become the most widely used broncodilators offering significantly improved beta-2 stimulation selectivity with fewer side-effects than previous bronchodilators.

Sweden's Sune K. Bergstrom and Bengt I. Samuelsson

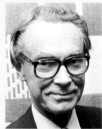

and Britain's John R. Vane are awarded the Nobel Prize in Medicine for their discoveries concerning "**prostaglandins** and related biologically active substances." First characterized nearly 50 years earlier by Bergstrom, prostaglandins and leukotrienes are found to play a crucial role in asthma and other inflammatory diseases.

1983

Joel Cooper, M.D., a transplant surgeon at Toronto General Hospital, performs the world's **first successful lung transplant** on a man dying of pulmonary fibrosis. This feat is followed in 1986 by the first successful double-lung transplant and in 1993 by a living related lung transplant in which lobes are donated by both the mother and father to their child.

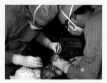

mid- 1980s

Vasodilators are used to treat pulmonary hypertension. It is subsequently learned that these drugs prolong life, improve exercise tolerance, and appear to reverse vascular structural changes in this lung disease.

MARCH 11, 1985
Mikhail Gorbachev becomes the leader of the U.S.S.R.

NOVEMBER 10, 1989
Celebrating Germans begin to tear down the Berlin Wall after East Germany opens its checkpoints to travel.

1985

Techniques employing **cell and molecular biology** are increasingly applied to the study of lung diseases.

After decades of decline, **tuberculosis** cases in the United States once again begin to rise. The onset of multi-drug-resistant strains, increased immigration from countries with high tuberculosis rates, and the impact of the HIV virus are all considered to contribute to the reversal.

Pulmonary rehabilitation is developed and recognized as important for patients with severe lung disease, especially chronic obstructive pulmonary disease (COPD).

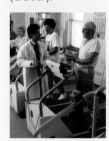

1986

Researchers first identify the role of **T-helper 1 (TH1)**

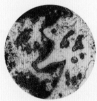

and T-helper 2 (TH2) in directing different immune-response pathways. TH1 cells are found to control cellular-immunity pathways in the fight against viruses and other intracellular pathogens, while TH2 cells control humoral immunity and up-regulate antibody production to fight extracellular organisms.

late 1980s

Researchers Anika and Lauri Laitinen (a husband and wife team from Helsinki) and Jean Bousquet from Montpellier **recognize asthma to be an inflammatory disease**, leading to the understanding by Barry Kay and C. J. Corrigan from London that T lymphocytes play a key role in regulating this inflammatory response through the elaboration of cytokines such as IL-4, IL-5 and IFN-gamma.

1989

Three teams of investigators from the Mayo Clinic, the University of Toronto, and Hadassah University Hospital in Jerusalem who were studying the long arm of chromosome 7 identify the gene associated with the development of **cystic fibrosis**. The gene is named "cystic fibrosis transmembrane conductance regulator."

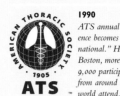

1990
ATS annual conference becomes "international." Held in Boston, more than 9,000 participants from around the world attend.

1989

High-resolution computed tomography (CT)

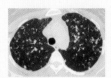

scanning is put into practice. This technique has transformed the clinical classification and diagnostic evaluation of diseases of the lung parenchyma.

1990s

Video-assisted thoracoscopy (VAT) allows surgeons access to all areas of the intrathoracic cavity while significantly limiting chest-wall trauma, deformity, and post-operative pain.

Directly observed therapy (DOT), in which tuberculosis patients are observed taking their medication, is shown to reduce the spread of the disease by improving compliance with drug regimens.

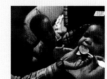

Adequate nutrition is recognized as important in maintaining ventilatory function in patients with **chronic obstructive pulmonary disease (COPD)**.

1990

Ten years of effort by the American Thoracic Society and others results in the reauthorization and **expansion of the federal Clean Air Act**. It lists 189 toxic air pollutants for which the Environmental Protection Agency will develop control technology standards to reduce the risk of cancer and other diseases resulting from exposure to these emissions.

1992

Wayne McLaren, a former professional rodeo rider and longtime smoker who became a "Marlboro Man" advertising Marlboro cigarettes, dies of lung cancer at the age of 51. Before his

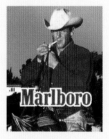

death, he films an anti-smoking television commercial, appears before the Massachusetts legislature in support of increased cigarette taxes, and meets with Philip Morris stockholders to urge limits on cigarette advertising.

MAY 10, 1994
Nelson Mandela is elected president in South Africa's first multiracial election.

JULY 5, 1996
Dolly the sheep, the first mammal to be successfully cloned from an adult cell, is born.

1993

A landmark study by Terry Young and others shows there is a high prevalence of **obstructive sleep apnea (OSA)** in the general population. This first major epidemiologic study on OSA establishes the public health burden of sleep-disordered breathing by concluding that as many as 4 percent of women and 9 percent of men suffer from this problem.

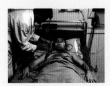

1994

Based upon a procedure developed by Otto Brantigan in

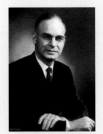

the 1950s, Joel Cooper performs **lung volume reduction surgery**, a treatment for patients with severe emphysema. It involves removing 20–30 percent of the lung tissues most damaged by the disease, giving the remaining, less diseased portion more room to function and resulting in easier breathing.

Brazilian researchers develop a unique approach to manage the frequently deadly **Acute Respiratory Distress Syndrome (ARDS)**: mechanical ventilation with low tidal volumes resulting in hypercapnia. In a multi-center, National Institutes of Health-sponsored clinical trial, this approach is later shown to reduce mortality.

1995

The American Thoracic Society releases a set of guidelines describing **optimum treatment for COPD**, a disease whose toll grows with each passing year.

Researchers identify **factor V Leiden**, a genetic mutation of the clotting factor V molecule that renders the molecule insensitive to activated protein C, a natural anticoagulant. This and other factors are subsequently shown to be associated with venous thrombosis, pulmonary embolism, and other conditions.

1996

The American Thoracic Society and American Lung Association release a **"Framework for Health Care Policy in the United States."** This position statement, noting that nearly 40 million Americans lack health insurance, urges the U.S. health care system to provide universal access to quality medical care in the most cost-effective manner.

2000
The American Thoracic Society and the American Lung Association become separate organizations.

ATS

SEPTEMBER 11, 2001
Terrorists fly hijacked planes into the U.S. World Trade Center, the Pentagon, and a field in Pennsylvania.

1997

The Institute of Medicine releases a ground-breaking report, **"Approaching Death: Improving Care at the End of Life."** The report

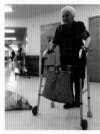

urges physicians to turn from aggressive conventional care of patients in their final phase of life to care which stresses comfort and quality of life. This new "end of life care" focus becomes an important component of the practice of critical care medicine.

2000s

Eliot Phillipson and his co-investigators determine that obstructive **sleep apnea is a significant contributor to sustained hypertension**, among the first studies showing cardiovascular interactions in sleep-disordered breathing. Subsequent studies, controlling for many other factors, have continued to support this strong link.

Researchers determine that lung injury may follow **inhalation of ozone, nitrogen dioxide, and other oxidants** from the atmosphere.

Researchers studying **innate immunity** in humans identify the presence of toll-like receptors, an evolutionarily conserved family of cell-surface molecules that participate in innate immune recognition of pathogen-associated molecular patterns.

Two groups of researchers—one representing the International Primary Pulmonary Hypertension Consortium and the other from Columbia University—discover the **genetic cause of familial primary pulmonary hypertension**: mutations in a gene (BMPR2) encoding a receptor that sits on the surface of a cell. Binding extracellular molecules, the receptor triggers changes in the cell's interior that affect cell behavior, including proliferation.

2001

The **Global Initiative for Asthma (GINA)** unveils a set of comprehensive guidelines for diagnosis and treatment of asthma, which is resurgent in much of the world.

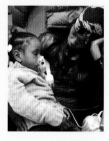

2005
ATS celebrates its 100th anniversary. The Society has more than 13,000 members worldwide.

2003

Researchers study the **effects of exposure to dust** released by the collapse of the World Trade Center twin towers on the lung function of New York City firefighters. Several related studies are published in the American Thoracic Society's official journal, the *American Journal of Respiratory and Critical Care Medicine*, in the months and years that follow.

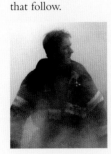

The quick spread of SARS from rural China to Hong

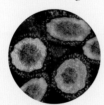

Kong and then across the world to Toronto demonstrates the **threat of new pandemics in the "global village."** The quick response of the World Health Organization, hospitals, and local public-health networks to contain the outbreak, however, also demonstrates the crucial nature of international cooperation to combat emerging diseases—as well as ones that have been known for millennia.

Results from the **National Emphysema Treatment Trial (NETT)** study on lung volume reduction surgery are presented at the American Thoracic Society's 2003 International Conference. The results conclude that selected patients with emphysema can benefit from the surgery.

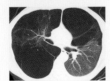

The American Thoracic Society convenes a workshop on the **"Ethical Principles of Critical Care"** to discuss and develop guidelines to assist investigators, regulatory agencies, clinicians, patients, and families in the ethical conduct of clinical research involving critically ill subjects.

2004

The American Thoracic Society publishes an updated statement on the **"Diagnosis and Initial Management of Nonmalignant Diseases Related to Asbestos."** The new statement estimates that asbestos is still a hazard for 1.3 million workers in the U.S. Also in 2004, the Society partners with the European Respiratory Society and releases updated chronic obstructive pulmonary disease (COPD) guidelines in an innovative, web-based publication, complete with a comprehensive patient education section.

2005

As this book was completed in 2004, it was impossible to predict the nature of the new discoveries to be reported in 2005. However, it is a safe prediction that the new year will bring continued advancements in pulmonary research and medicine and that as the American Thoracic Society begins its second century of fighting lung disease, it will continue in its work to create collaboration, foster innovation, and further understanding among the world's lung disease and critical care experts.

TUBERCULOSIS

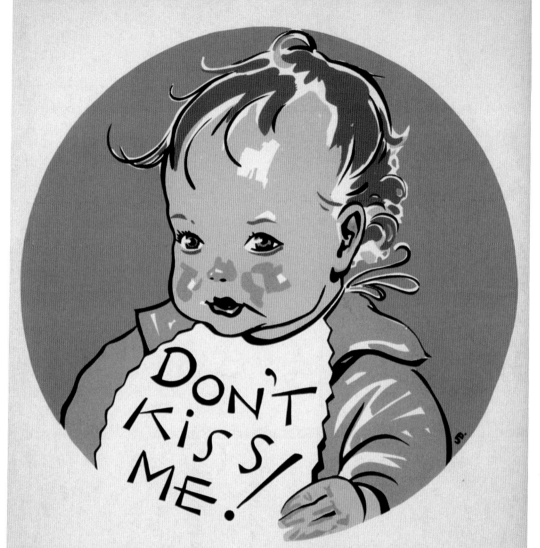

YOUR KISS OF AFFECTION THE GERM OF INFECTION

TOWN OF HEMPSTEAD, W.H. RUNCIE MD. HEALTH OFFICER
WPA FEDERAL ART PROJECT DISTRICT 4

CHAPTER FOUR

Public Health, Public Service

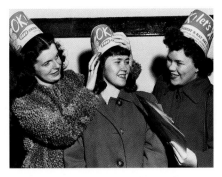

The more innovative the publicity, the more people would listen. College students in 1947 doffed "high hats" to publicize a public-health initiative to identify individuals with tuberculosis via widespread use of X-rays.

"The awareness that health is dependent upon habits that we control makes us the first generation in history that to a large extent determines its own destiny."

—JIMMY CARTER, THIRTY-NINTH U.S. PRESIDENT (1924–PRESENT)

Aᴳᴬᴵᴺ ᴬᴺᴰ ᴬᴳᴬᴵᴺ during the history of respiratory medicine, one question keeps arising: Why did it take so long for governments to assume a leading role in improving public health?

As early as 1916, the National Tuberculosis Association (NTA) and the American Sanatorium Association (forerunner of the American Thoracic Society) adopted a resolution declaring that federal government leadership in tuberculosis control was "desirable and necessary," and that the "proper federal agency for the purpose is the U.S. Public Health Service." But federal government efforts in the United States and abroad remained nearly nonexistent, and the U.S. Public Health Service division of tuberculosis was not created until 1944.

Few called on the government to do more. A few writers, such as Frank Norris in his famous novels *The Octopus* and *The Pit,* decried the dehumanizing effects of the industrial world, and Charlie Chaplin satirized them in his 1936 movie *Modern Times.* Yet no one seemed to realize that by forcing industry to humanize the workplace and improve living conditions, lawmakers could slow the tuberculosis epidemic's seemingly inexorable progress.

Tuberculosis was not the only disease or condition whose occupational causes were well known to government and industry alike. As long as miners have been digging out gold and coal from underground veins, they've dreaded "miner's lung," the condition that, years after exposure, caused their lungs to become inflamed and scarred. Hippocrates mentioned the condition over two thousand years ago, and it was the focus of Paracelsus's mid-sixteenth century book *On The Miner's Sickness.* Though the specific causes of silicosis, asbestosis, black lung, and other "miner's

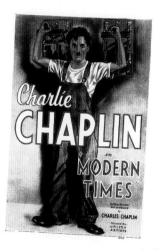

In his classic, *Modern Times,* Charlie Chaplin pokes fun at the dehumanizing effects of the industrial production line. But the fight to make the workplace safer—and less of a disease reservoir—was deadly serious.

Opposite: Public education has always gone hand-in-hand with the fight against respiratory disease. This poster, originally published circa 1940, sought to reduce the incidence of tuberculosis.

sicknesses" were identified only relatively recently, no one ever doubted that they came from working in the mines. Yet for generations, nothing was done to protect the miners and their families.

The inaction extended to many other diseases with recognized environmental or occupational causes, including mesothelioma, lung cancer, emphysema, asthma, and chronic obstructive pulmonary disease (COPD). All have killed thousands of people in the past century alone. Yet it was not until 1964, with the release of the seminal *Surgeon General's Report on Smoking and Health,* that the U.S. government finally took on an aggressive public-health role, joining medical professionals and educators to confront smoking, a major cause of many preventable diseases. And once again, as they had with the tuberculosis epidemic, the American Thoracic Society helped goad the government into action.

The Surgeon General's Report and Public-health Advocacy

Although nicotine's addictive properties were not acknowledged by the Surgeon General's Office until the 1980s, other observers have known about tobacco addiction for centuries.

In the early sixteenth century, a Spanish missionary named Bartolomé de las Casas noted that South American Indians used tobacco habitually, and seemed unable to stop. What he didn't mention was that the habit had been spread by the Spanish themselves. Until the conquest, historian Johannes Wilbert points out, tobacco in the New World seems to have been used exclusively in rituals and for medicinal purposes. Once the Spanish started using it recreationally, he explains, "the ideological tenets of tobacco beliefs began to shift increasingly from the religious to the profane" among the Indians as well.

Less than a century later, the habit had spread so widely in Europe that King James I of England wrote "A Counterblaste to Tobacco," in which he called the leaf "bewitching" to its users, as essential to them as sleep.

It didn't take very long before experts identified nicotine as the culprit within the leaf. In the 1850s, a poem in *Harper's Weekly* magazine made a play on words with "Old Nick" (the devil) and the "nic" found in tobacco. "Dulls the sense, defiles the breath," the poem said of smoking. "Depraves the taste, depletes the purse;/Poisons the very air with death." The slang phrase "coffin nails" to describe cigarettes came into vogue at around the same time.

Just as they did with tuberculosis, hucksters of all sorts recognized tobacco addiction's money-making potential. Advertisements for tobacco cures were everywhere, including one called Baco-Curo that claimed to drain the nicotine from your system even as you smoked. By the end of

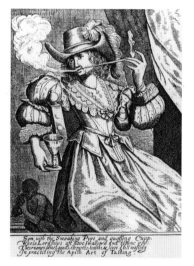

The Evil Weed. In this 1660 image, a "gentlewoman" smokes a long-stemmed pipe. Almost as soon as tobacco came to the Old World, education efforts sprang up to convince the public that the habit was unpleasant and unhealthy. For centuries, however, such efforts were almost uniformly unsuccessful.

the nineteenth century, an enterprising doctor named Leslie Keeley had opened two hundred Keeley Institutes across the country, offering "cures" for alcohol, opium, or tobacco addiction with injections of "double chloride of gold."

Early in the twentieth century, concern over cigarette smoking had grown serious enough that some states temporarily banned their sale, as did the U.S. Navy. The federal Pure Food and Drug Act of 1906 listed nicotine as a drug, although it was removed from the list after an early showing of tobacco-industry clout in Washington. By the time of World War I, however, the armed forces not only approved of cigarettes, they distributed them for free among those in the services. They felt that cigarettes were the least of several evils; those who smoked, the theory went, were less likely to drink and consort with loose women.

As scientific studies made the causal link between smoking and lung cancer and other respiratory diseases increasingly clear, the public wasn't listening. By the mid-1950s more than half of all American men smoked cigarettes and at least a third of American women had the habit. As alcohol prohibition had proven thirty years earlier, merely banning tobacco was doomed to fail. Another method of getting the public's attention was needed to change the deeply ingrained habit.

The solution was to bring together medical science, public education, and government action in a unique and powerful manner. In the late 1950s the American Thoracic Society began to scientifically document smoking's effects on health. The goal was to provide undeniable scientific basis for any antismoking statements and programs that the National Tuberculosis and Respiratory Disease Association (NTRDA), precursor to the American Lung Association, might develop.

In 1960 the NTRDA adopted the American Thoracic Society's first official findings on the topic. These findings stated unequivocally that smoking was a major cause of lung cancer and that "recent studies show that cigarette smoking is a factor in such crippling lung diseases as chronic bronchitis and emphysema." The statement then called upon parents, teachers, and physicians to make sure young people understood these facts before starting to smoke.

By 1962 a groundswell for governmental action against smoking was gaining momentum. Under orders from President John F. Kennedy, Surgeon General Luther Terry convened a committee of experts to conduct a comprehensive review of the scientific literature on smoking.

The members of the committee were nominated by the NTRDA, the American Cancer Society, the American Medical Association, and other groups. Those finally chosen were experts in the fields of medicine, surgery, pharmacology, and statistics—and included only individuals who had taken no previous public stand on tobacco use. For over a year the

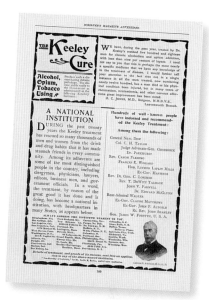

The Keeley Cure, a 1904 elixir that supposedly ended addictions to tobacco, opium, and other substances, was just one of countless potions that promised a painless way to kick a variety of habits. This one was undoubtedly no more successful than those that came before and after.

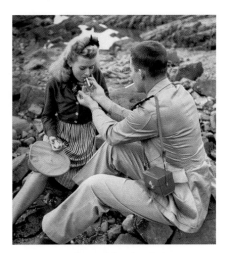

A U.S. navy pilot and his date light up in this World War II image. Though the military at the time didn't exactly approve of smoking, it considered tobacco a lesser evil than alcohol or consorting with the wrong kind of women, and therefore didn't actively discourage the habit.

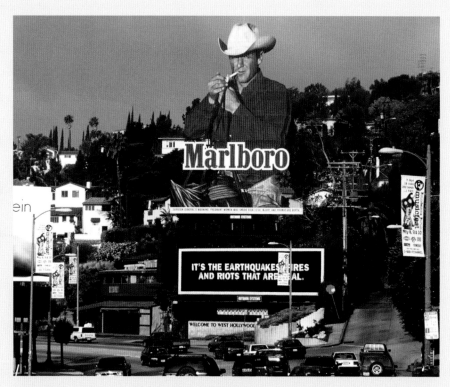

A landmark in American advertising history, the Marlboro Man has also become a symbol of how even the mighty cowboy can be laid low by the dire health effects of cigarette smoking.

Smoking and Advertising:
Slick Shtick for the Cancer Stick

The understanding that cigarette smoking is harmful to one's health did not begin with the 1964 Surgeon General's Report, or even with the research by American Thoracic Society scientists that laid the groundwork for the report. Almost as soon as cigarettes became big business in Europe and the United States in the early twentieth century, the tobacco companies began to fight the perception that smoking was an unhealthy, unclean, dangerous habit— a perception reflected in such popular descriptive terms for cigarettes as "coffin nails," "wheezers," and "lung dusters." Nor did it help when such prominent heroes of industry as Henry Ford and Thomas Edison railed against cigarette smoking.

Rather than ignoring such pejoratives, the cigarette companies (while simultaneously trying to make cigarettes seem stylish, even glamorous) used the health concerns as hammers to bludgeon each other in advertising. Chesterfield had perhaps the simplest blanket defense of its product: its cigarettes, ads read, "Cause no ills."

Other advertisements took a slightly more complex route. Old Gold had "Not a cough in a carload." Camels boasted, "Not a single case of throat irritation." Philip Morris pointed out that "Smoking's more fun when you're not worried by throat irritation or smoker's cough." Overall, as *BusinessWeek* magazine pointed out in 1953, the cigarette companies seemed determined to get people to smoke by "screaming at the top of their lungs about nicotine, cigarette hangovers, smoker's cough, mildness, and kindred subjects."

Occasionally, the companies tried another tack: touting the health benefits of smoking, such as improved concentration, relaxation, and weight loss. But even here, health issues remained simmering below the surface. One ad touted the "strong nerves" that cigarettes provided to lung surgeons! Another suggested that Americans forgo fattening candy, so bad for your health, and "Reach for a Lucky instead of a sweet." (Outraged candy manufacturers pointed out that while sweets might contain calories, cigarettes "poison with nicotine every organ of your body.")

Even today, decades after the Surgeon General's Report and in an era when smoking is increasingly restricted, cigarette companies still use a health subtext in much of their advertising. "Alive with Pleasure!" trumpets Newport's longtime slogan. Note that the words *"pleasure"* and *"alive"* get the same emphasis. Cigarette advertising has not come that far from "Cause no ills."

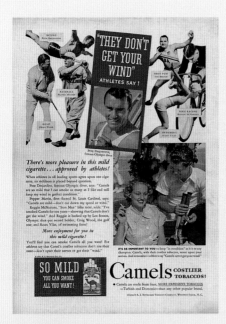

From the earliest days of cigarette smoking, questions about tobacco's possible ill effects were widespread. In response, cigarette companies each vied to claim that their brands were the least destructive to smokers' health.

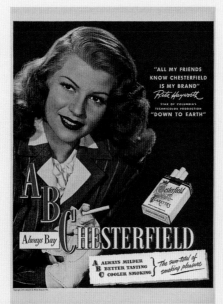

The subtext of cigarette advertisements was often plain. This one said that if you smoked Chesterfield, you too could be as glamorous as Rita Hayworth.

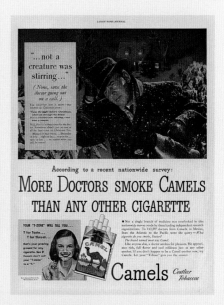

This ad relied on "logic," asking how Camels could be unhealthy if doctors smoked them.

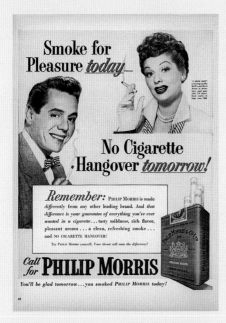

And this one combined the two approaches, saying that your life could be as riotous and entertaining as Lucille Ball and Desi Arnaz's if you smoked Philip Morris...yet you wouldn't regret it in the morning.

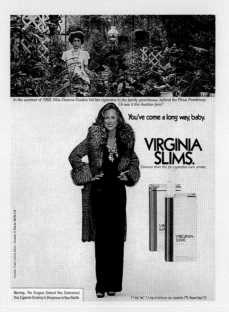

As soon as cigarette smoking became an acceptable habit among women, the tobacco companies were there to flatter—and capture—the burgeoning new market.

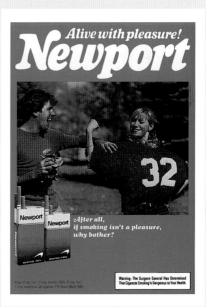

Today's cigarette advertisements differ little from older ones. Smoke Newport, this one says, and not only will your existence be filled with pleasure, but you'll stay alive.

members reviewed more than seven thousand scientific articles and met with more than 150 consultants.

Luther Terry released his report on January 11, 1964, choosing a Saturday to minimize the effect on the stock market and maximize the news impact in the Sunday papers. The report could not have been more unequivocal: Smoking, it said, was responsible for a seventy percent increase in mortality of smokers over nonsmokers; increased the risk of lung cancer ten to twenty times; was the most important cause of chronic bronchitis; and was associated with increased rates of emphysema and coronary heart disease.

The Surgeon General's Report on Smoking and Health "hit the country like a bombshell," Terry recalled later. "It was front page news and a lead story on every radio and television station in the United States and many abroad." It also had a lasting impact: surveys showed that while in 1958 less than half of Americans believed that smoking caused lung cancer, by 1968 nearly eighty percent did.

But the report and follow-up publicity campaigns by the NTRDA and others didn't end the battle against smoking. It was just beginning. Through the Tobacco Institute, tobacco companies immediately sought to discredit the report's findings.

Less than three weeks after the report was issued, a confidential memo to Philip Morris's CEO from its president George Weissman called the report a "propaganda blast," and said that the company must "provide some answers which will give smokers a psychological crutch and self-rationale to continue smoking." He even suggested that company officials contact "all the cartoonists, television gag writers, satirical reviews, etc., to apply the light touch to this question."

The years that followed saw an ongoing conflict between the enormous financial resources of the cigarette companies and the cooperative efforts of the federal government and health organizations. To counteract the cigarette companies' relentless waves of propaganda, a series of government reports, including *Health Consequences of Smoking* (1969), *Health Consequences of Smoking for Women* (1980), and *Health Consequences of Involuntary Smoking* (1986), expanded on the findings of the original Surgeon General's Report. Simultaneously, the members of the American Thoracic Society provided the clinical and scientific backing for a series of ambitious antismoking public-education efforts.

David Burns, M.D., of the University of California at San Diego, was the chief author or scientific editor of many of the reports that followed the original 1964 report, including crucial early findings on second-hand smoke. One of his important focuses has been the cigarette companies' ongoing attempts to convince smokers that "reduced yield" (low nicotine) cigarettes are healthier than traditional ones. "It's a fraud," he says. "We've discovered that the amount of nicotine ingested doesn't vary

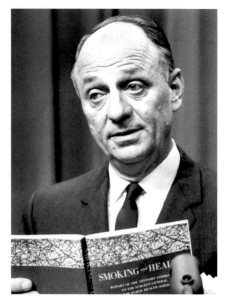

Surgeon General Luther L. Terry at the press conference announcing the release of his 1964 report on smoking and health. The report (based partly on important research by the American Thoracic Society) created a bombshell in the United States, leading to the first strong antismoking laws.

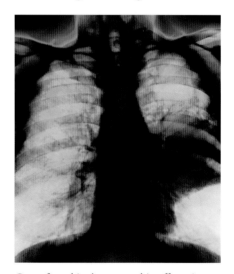

One of smoking's catastrophic effects: image of a cancerous lung. The black and orange coloration in the middle of the lung shows where lung cancer has already made its devastating mark.

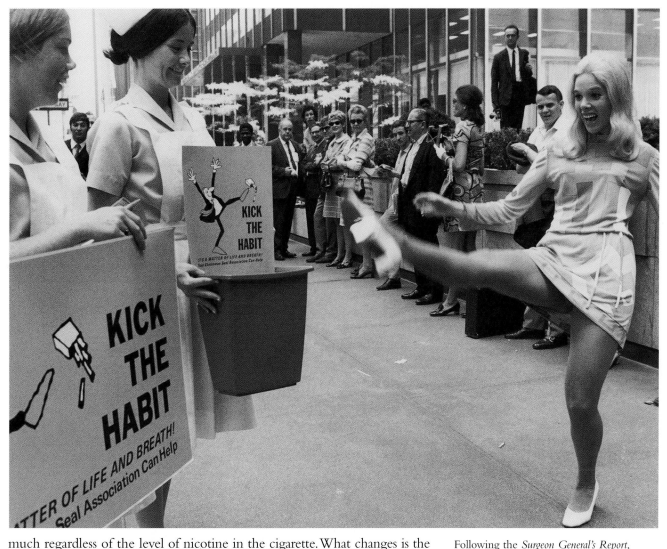

much regardless of the level of nicotine in the cigarette. What changes is the way you smoke the cigarette."

Researchers have found that receptors in the pharynx are susceptible to nicotine. "These receptors communicate to the brain when you're not getting enough nicotine," Burns explains. "So you customize the way you smoke to preserve the dose you need."

The four decades since the 1964 Surgeon General's Report have proven something about the three-pronged approach utilizing science, education, and legislation: It works. Smoking rates, even among teens—a long holdout against downward smoking trends—have been on the decline in recent years. The American Thoracic Society and others have helped lead efforts resulting in nationwide smoking-cessation initiatives; health-education programs on smoking during pregnancy; a smoking ban on airline flights and in most workplaces; and a wide variety of other antismoking laws and regulations. Though the battle continues, this approach has proven to be a far more successful one than any that came before, and one that has since been used to address many other environmental and occupational threats.

Following the *Surgeon General's Report*, antismoking efforts redoubled across the United States. This 1970 image shows the "kickoff" of a New York City campaign, just one of the many that helped lead to a gradual decline in smoking rates.

The Government versus Respiratory Disease

Even before the antismoking battle took center stage in the early 1960s, the American Thoracic Society, NTRDA, American Heart Association, and other groups selected additional respiratory-health issues to raise. In an age when cities were often choked with smog, no issue was more pertinent—or more urgent—than air pollution.

In 1956 the American Thoracic Society sought to give the NTRDA the scientific evidence it needed to focus on respiratory diseases caused by air pollution—and to begin strengthening links with federal programs as well. "Air pollution: little is known as to public health significance," read the NTRDA's guidelines for new activities in 1959. "[Explore] cooperative action with U.S. Public Health Service to determine relationship between air pollution and disease; control of air pollution might then become a major goal of the NTRDA." Research from American Thoracic Society's members would eventually provide an unbreakable link between airborne pollutants and such diseases as asthma, bronchitis and others. By providing strong scientific evidence of air pollution's dangerous effects (especially on children), the NTRDA, the Society, and other organizations were able to unleash a strong effort to pressure the federal government to control pollutants at their sources.

In its first foray into legislative lobbying outside of tuberculosis, in 1961 the NTRDA supported federal legislation on air pollution and urged the Public Health Service to wage an all-out war on respiratory diseases resulting from environmental hazards. By 1965, the NTRDA was devoting an entire issue of its *Bulletin* to air pollution—and the Public Health Service was ordering twenty thousand copies to distribute. This was followed by the formation of the National Air Conservation Commission in 1966, with an avowed goal of seeing federal air pollution control legislation passed.

In conjunction with ongoing research detailing the respiratory effects of airborne pollutants and such public-education efforts as "Cleaner Air Week," these intensifying lobbying efforts brought pressure on the federal government that would have been unheard of a generation earlier. The result was one of the landmark laws in U.S. history: the Clean Air Act of 1970.

In earlier acts in 1963 and 1967, the federal government had supported states in their attempts to quantify the effects of air pollution. But the 1970 Clean Air Act, recognizing that air pollution obeyed no state boundaries, established a complex set of rules governing issues from acid rain to ozone depletion and pollution sources from lawn mowers to nuclear power plants. It marked the first time that the government sought to protect the health of its citizens through a wide-ranging set of environmental standards.

But the passage of the Clean Air Act marked the beginning of the battle, not the end. Politicians and industries alike have repeatedly endeavored

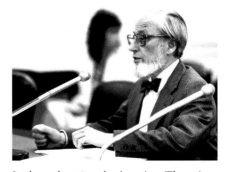

In the early 1980s, the American Thoracic Society expanded its role in public health. Testifying before Congress here is the Society's 1986 president Gordon Snider, just one of many members who have provided vital information to the federal government on many issues, including the role of environmental pollutants in asthma and COPD.

Opposite: The U.S. Capitol shrouded in smog on a typical Washington summer morning. Through its expert testimony in Congress, the American Thoracic Society has helped shape many anti-pollution laws.

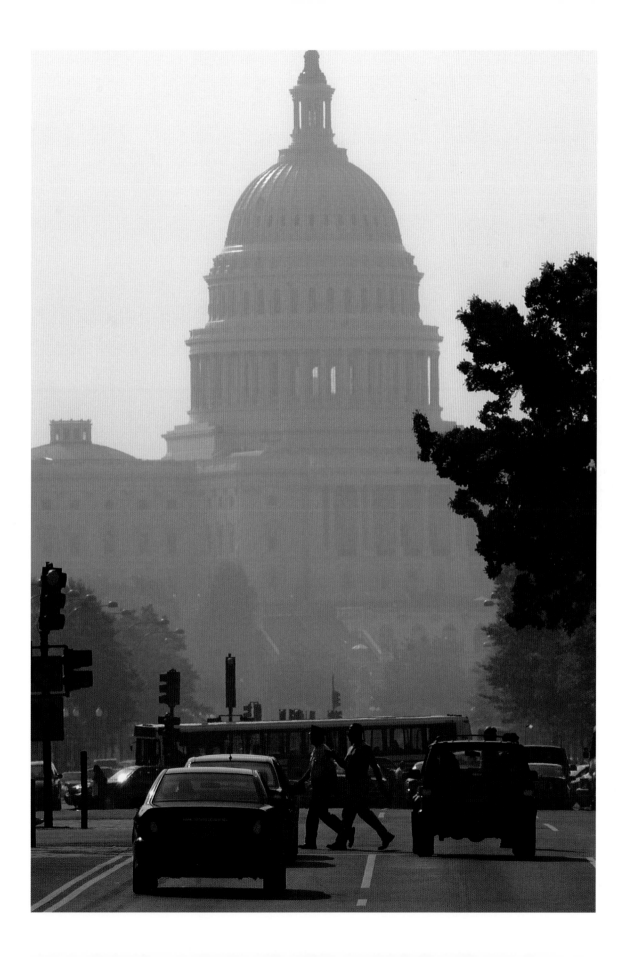

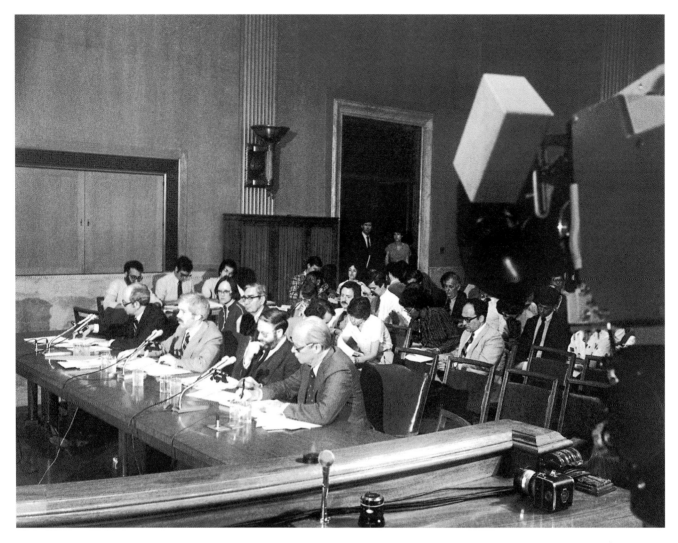

to weaken it, and those in favor of maintaining or strengthening the Act have increasingly come to rely on the American Thoracic Society and other organizations to provide supporting expertise.

In 1980, the American Lung Association/American Thoracic Society opened an office in Washington, D.C., with the stated priority of lobbying for increased tuberculosis funding and reauthorization of the Clean Air Act. To lend the essential scientific knowledge, the American Thoracic Society's Assembly on Environmental and Occupational Health, under John O'Neil's leadership, immediately put together a roster of experts on the health effects of air pollution. The goal was to communicate to Congress the need to strengthen and extend the Clean Air Act.

Future American Thoracic Society president Homer Boushey, Jr., M.D., expressed that need when he testified before Congress in 1981. His testimony, given to the Senate Committee on Environment and Public Works, presented cutting-edge research on the adverse effects on sulfur dioxide on asthmatic patients, while also stressing the role of the Act's Ambient Air Quality Standards in reducing levels of this and other pollutants.

The dawn of a new age: American Thoracic Society members testify before the Senate Committee on Environment and Public Works over reauthorization of the Clean Air Act in June, 1981. This marked the onset of the Society's long-term commitment to influencing public policy on air pollution, mine safety, and other issues.

Boushey pointed out that the Air Quality Standards separated the costs of pollution abatement from identification of adverse health effects. "This ensures that we first determine what air pollution does to health before we determine how rapidly and at what cost we pursue our health objective," he commented.

At heart, this simple sentence defines what has made the Clean Air Act so controversial: it flies in the face of the belief that respiratory health should be subjected to cost-benefit analysis; that, in fact, it is easier to treat the patient made ill by air pollution than to clean up the air.

After nearly ten years of testimony by American Thoracic Society members and countless others, in 1990 the revised Clean Air Act tightened emission standards for power plants and strengthened other aspects of the Act. Since then, however, shifting political winds have repeatedly threatened to reverse the gains of recent years, which include the steady decline of such pollutants as carbon monoxide, nitrogen dioxide, sulfur dioxide, and lead within the United States.

The American Thoracic Society has continued to take a strong role in challenging the government to continue addressing air-pollution issues. In a 1999 statement, the organization pointed out that "the health effects of outdoor air pollution remain a public-health concern in developing and developed countries alike," with levels of diseases such as asthma and COPD continuing to rise. Further, focusing on a crucial but often neglected factor in the debate, the 1999 statement said, "The formalization of the concept of environmental justice acknowledges that the effects of specific pollutants cannot be evaluated in isolation without giving consideration to the over-lapping exposures of populations, often minority group members of low socioeconomic status, who live in neighborhoods that are heavily exposed to multiple environmental contaminants."

American Thoracic Society members also continue to serve as expert witnesses as Congress debates new air-pollution measures. In one 2003 session before the House Subcommittee on Veterans Affairs, Housing, and Urban Development, the Society was represented by David J. Tollerud, M.D., M.P.H. "It is estimated that 141 million Americans live in areas that expose them to unsafe levels of ozone or particulate matter," Tollerud said. "That means half of America is breathing polluted air."

In his wide-ranging testimony, Tollerud described the scientific evidence proving, in his words, why "exposure to polluted air matters." He also challenged Congress to increase funding for the Environmental Protection Agency (EPA); urged the EPA to enforce 1997 rules governing fine particulate and ozone levels; expressed the American Thoracic Society's deep concern over recent efforts to revise New Source Review provisions for airborne pollutants; and recommended increasing the budget of the EPA's Asthma Research programs.

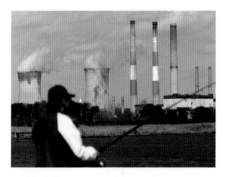

In a nation that has to balance industry with the environment, air quality with energy production, the American Thoracic Society has sought to protect the respiratory health of Americans through medical research and public policy alike.

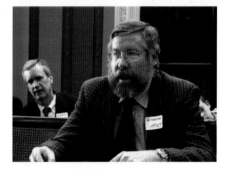

Dr. David J. Tollerud, Chair of the American Thoracic Society Assembly on Environmental and Occupational Health, testifies on air pollution issues before a House Subcommittee on Veterans Affairs, Housing, and Urban Development.

Following pages: A worldwide problem: This photograph from space reveals the glow caused by air pollution that sits over the Indian Ocean. While many of the American Thoracic Society's legislative efforts have focused on the United States, a global focus has become increasingly prominent in recent years.

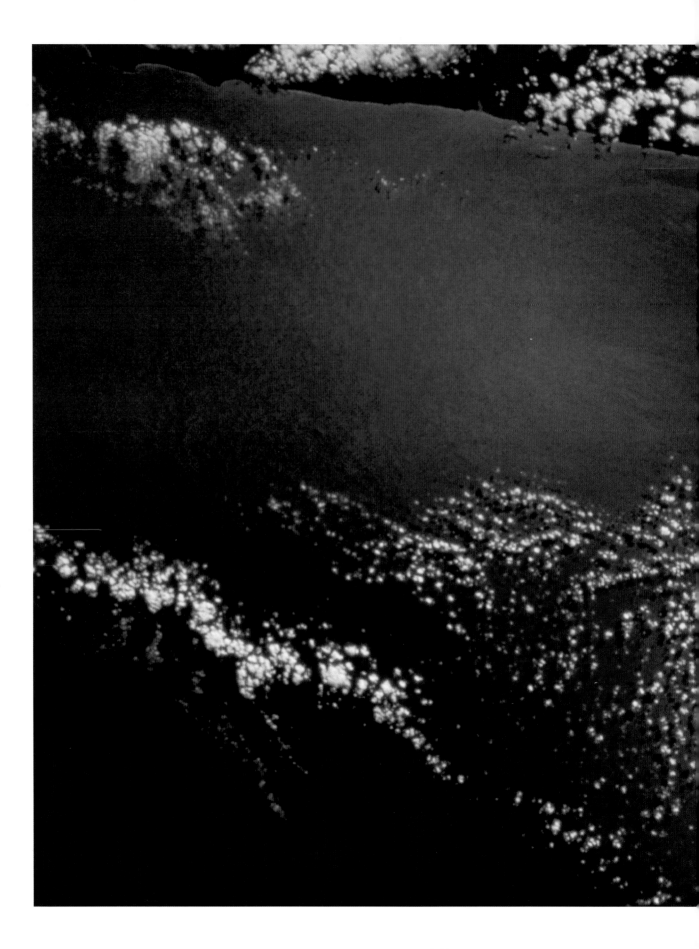

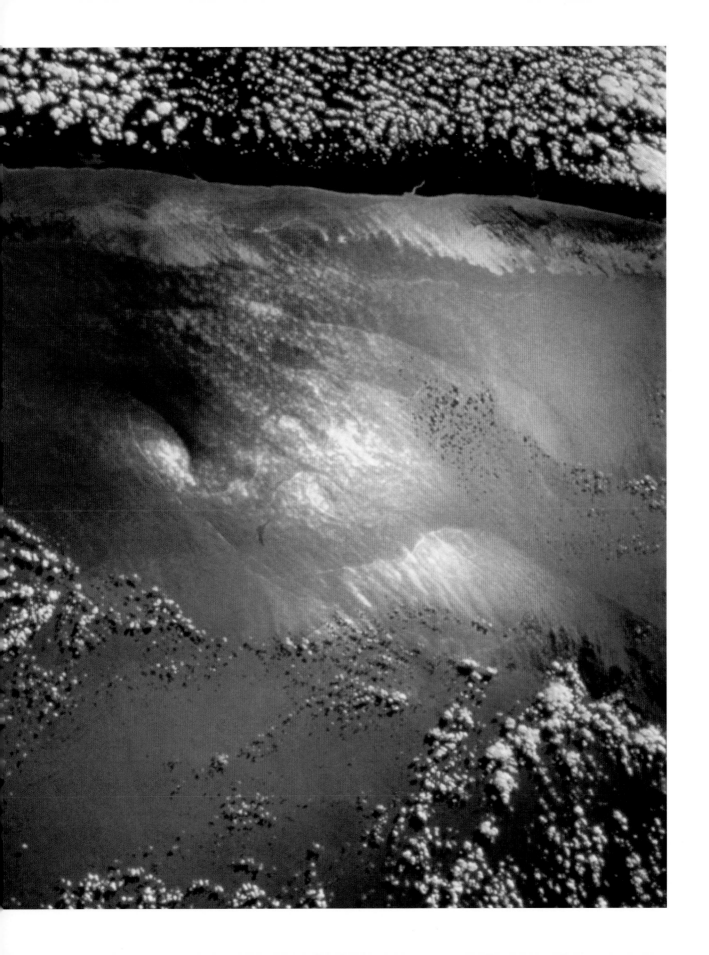

In addition to passing the Clean Air Act of 1970, the federal government addressed a variety of other issues with respiratory-health implications. The creation of the Occupational Safety and Health Act and the Environmental Protection Agency in 1970 and the passage of the Mine Safety Act of 1977 confronted the fact that respiratory disease is a national issue requiring programs on a scale that matches the threat. Yet these efforts have also had to withstand repeated attacks from industry and others, while the diseases they aim to prevent continue to take an enormous toll.

Silica, Asbestos, and Occupational Lung Disease

The severe health effects of exposure to silica and asbestos have been known for centuries. Today, after the passage of the Mine Safety Act, the establishment of the Mine Safety and Health Administration, and other federal efforts, a range of laws seek to protect workers and others from these hazardous minerals. Advocacy, publicity, and intense lobbying have succeeded in creating public awareness of the issues involved, but in mining towns, in car-repair shops, even in homes across the globe, the story of asbestos and silica exposure will continue to play out for decades to come. It is a striking story of medical professionals and government regulators backed by hard scientific evidence battling influential industries and corporations that have refused to acknowledge problems exist.

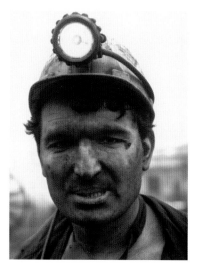

Coal-miners pneumoconiosis, better known as black-lung disease, has stricken countless miners for generations. Though laws regulating coal dust have reduced levels in U.S. mines, the disease remains endemic in much of the rest of the world.

The battle against occupational lung disease is far from won. "Despite all efforts to prevent it, this ancient disease still afflicts hundreds of thousands of miners and millions of other workers engaged in hazardous, dusty occupations in many countries," states the World Health Organization (WHO) in its "Global Programme on Elimination of Silicosis."

Among the WHO's recommendations are "laws and regulations, enforcement of occupational exposure limits and technical standards, governmental advisory services, an effective system of inspection, a well-organized reporting system, and a national action programme involving governmental agencies, industry, and trade unions." These, the organization points out, "are the necessary elements of a sound infrastructure which is required to combat silicosis successfully."

Yet the reality remains far from this ideal. In a 2004 hearing, Senator Harry Reid of Nevada revealed that the U.S. Department of Energy (DOE) had allowed workers to dig a tunnel in Yucca Mountain, which contains silica, without requiring them to wear protective gear. The Department then allegedly changed the results of silica-level tests to allow work to continue. "At best, DOE's actions are negligent and at worst criminal," said Reid, whose father was a miner who suffered from silicosis.

Reid and other Nevada officials had hoped to shut down work on the mine and also to establish a compensation fund for the affected

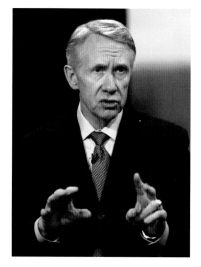

United States senator Harry Reid's father was a miner who suffered from silicosis. Today, Reid fights to reduce exposure to silica dust among the miners in his home state of Nevada and across the country.

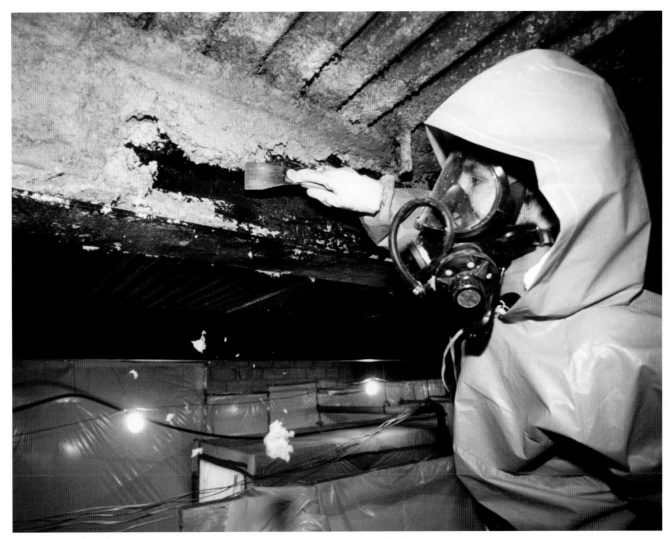

workers. As of this book's publication, however, such resolutions had not been achieved.

Asbestos's story is just as heartbreaking. "Asbestos was clearly bad stuff, and trying to regulate it was very contentious and fraught with all sorts of battles," former EPA administrator William Ruckelshaus told journalists Andrew Schneider and David McCumber for their book *The Air That Kills*. "EPA's scientists would reach a conclusion that supported the need for tighter controls or lower exposure levels or whatever. Then scientists hired by industry interests would often present a completely opposite interpretation of the same issue, showing, in their opinion, that tighter regulation wasn't needed. Sometimes it boiled down to who had more powerful friends."

Perhaps the most notorious example of this involves W. R. Grace's Zonolite vermiculite mine near Libby, Montana—a mine that along with vermiculite contained an abundance of tremolite, a rare, toxic form of asbestos. Grace ran Zonolite between 1963 and 1990, when he finally closed the mine. Currently, more than two hundred Libby residents have died of asbestos exposure and more than four hundred have been diagnosed with

Dangerous but legal. Despite irrefutable evidence that it causes cancer and other life-threatening lung diseases, asbestos is not banned in the United States. Every year, miners, builders, auto mechanics, and others are exposed to its severe health effects.

diseases caused by asbestos. Those affected include miners' family members, harmed by dust tracked back into the house by the mine workers.

The Environmental Protection Agency and the Occupational Safety and Health Administration have promulgated numerous laws and regulations governing asbestos exposure, abatement procedures, and other "public protection" acts. Remarkably, despite widespread belief that use of asbestos has been banned for home construction, automobile brakes, and other purposes, it remains available. In 1989 the EPA announced a ban, but the courts overturned it in 1991.

Today, the nation's hundreds of thousands of auto mechanics, home builders, and others still handle asbestos daily, often without realizing it or knowing about safety guidelines. And each year, at least thirty thousand new cases of asbestos-related cancer are diagnosed in the United States and Europe, along with many times that number of other asbestos-related diseases.

These cases, and the litigation that has surrounded asbestos for at least two decades, led the American Thoracic Society to lobby once again for increased funding for research and treatment of occupational lung disease. The Society has helped achieve budget increases for the National Institute of Occupational Safety and Health, while also working with unions and employers to set up basic research programs in occupational health as well as undertake program evaluations.

The American Thoracic Society's rigorous scientific approach has also aided countless physicians in diagnosing and treating asbestos-related disease. The Society's landmark 1986 *Diagnosis of Nonmalignant Diseases Related to Asbestos* provided a basis for diagnosis until 2004, when it was replaced by the Society's updated and far-reaching *Recommendations for the Diagnosis and Treatment of Non-Malignant Disease Caused by Asbestos Exposure.*

In joining basic scientific knowledge with a strongly held public posture, the Society has assumed a role that will be increasingly important in the years to come. As then-Society president Dr. Homer Boushey, Jr., put it in testimony before the Senate Judiciary Committee in 2003, "As physicians who diagnose, treat, and research asbestos-related conditions, we are . . . committed to ensuring that appropriate medical criteria are used and applied in whatever legislative proposals move forward."

Asthma and COPD: Growing Epidemics

In addition to occupational health reform, a quick glance at the programs for the American Thoracic Society's recent International Conferences reveals respiratory specialists' focus on asthma and chronic obstructive pulmonary disease (COPD), two respiratory diseases whose prevalence is growing each year.

Individual asbestos fibers are so small, they cannot be seen under a microscope until the lungs coat them with iron. Once coated, as above, they are referred to as ferruginous bodies and are often looked for in lung cells to prove exposure to asbestos.

ASTHMA

Asthma currently affects between seventeen and twenty million Americans, including four million children. Each year, it results in about five thousand deaths, two million emergency room visits, 14.5 million missed work-days, and 14 million missed school days. Asthma rates continue to climb every year, with children again at greatest risk: Prevalence rates between 1980 and 1996 climbed nearly 75 percent for children under the age of five.

The worldwide scenario is no brighter. At the fourth World Asthma Meeting, held in Bangkok, Thailand, in February 2004, experts estimated that three hundred million people now suffer from asthma worldwide. Many countries are seeing up to a 5 percent rise in cases each year, and the number is expected to reach 400 million by 2024.

In the United States, African Americans and other ethnic minorities suffer the highest prevalence of asthma. According to epidemiological research conducted by American Thoracic Society members, asthma-attack prevalence rates were a third higher among African Americans than Caucasians, and hospitalization rates were three times higher.

Many of the triggers of asthma are environmental, including such factors as allergens, cigarette smoke, ozone and other air pollutants, and chemicals. While respiratory syncytial virus (RSV) or other viral infections contracted early in life can contribute to later development of asthma, even in these cases there is a strong environmental component: maternal smoking, second-hand smoke, and lack of breastfeeding can be major factors in the prevalence and severity of childhood RSV.

But even though much remains to be learned to cure asthma, it should not disguise the extraordinary recent advances in understanding about the pathogenesis of the disease. Nor should it obscure the great strides made by physicians, scientists, and pharmaceutical companies in managing asthma. A disease that remained an untreatable mystery for centuries has revealed many of its secrets in just the past few decades.

Research in the 1960s by Margaret Becklake, professor emerita in the Department of Epidemiology and Biostatistics and Department of Medicine, McGill University, Montreal, and others, along with the development of bronchoscopy, bronchoalveolar lavage, airway biopsy, and measurement of airway gases have greatly improved our understanding of asthma pathogenesis. Though today the wisdom that asthma is, at heart, an inflammatory disease is widely held, it wasn't until 1997 that the National Heart, Lung, and Blood Institute (NHLBI) released a definition of asthma that revealed how much had been learned—and how quickly.

The NHLBI included the following features considered to be integral to the definition of asthma: recurrent episodes of respiratory symptoms; variable airflow obstruction that is often reversible, either spontaneously or

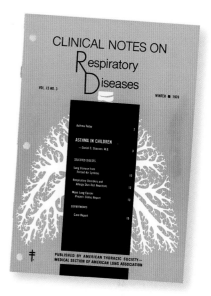

Asthma, a respiratory disease whose incidence continues to rise, has long been a major focus of research at the American Thoracic Society, as demonstrated by this 1976 Society publication focusing on the disease in children.

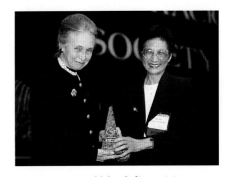

Dr. Margaret Becklake (left) receiving the 1997 American Thoracic Society Distinguished Achievement Award from Moira Chan-Yeung. Becklake's seminal work in the 1960s on asthma led to a profoundly deeper understanding of the pathogenesis of the once-mysterious disease.

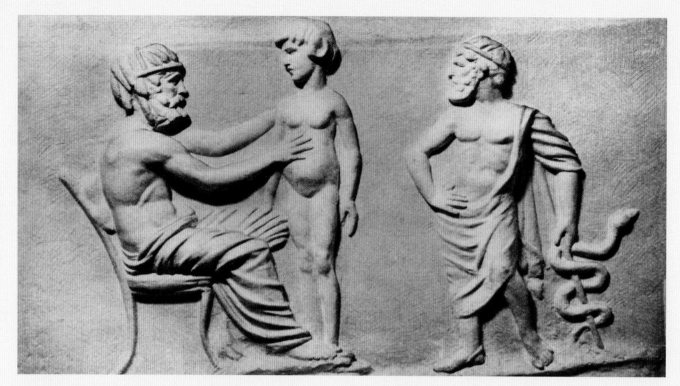

The great Hippocrates (the "Father of Medicine") looks on as a physician examines a young patient, in this bas-relief from about 350 B.C. Hippocrates and other early physicians knew of asthma, but coming up with a successful treatment was beyond their grasp.

Early Asthma Treatments

Symptoms resembling those of asthma were mentioned as long ago as 1550 B.C. in the Ebers papyrus from ancient Egypt. A similar condition was described in the earliest medical textbook, the Chinese Neu Ching, in about 1000 B.C. As early as 81 A.D., the ancient Greeks identified the symptoms and classified them as a disease.

Yet before the development of effective asthma therapies in the early 1900s, medical practitioners had to depend on a variety of creative, outlandish, and frequently hopeless potions while attempting to treat this chronic disease. Some of the most colorful—and a few with some actual efficacy—are described below:

- **Seeking a dry climate, avoiding sexual activity, and eating chicken soup.** This treatment regimen, advocated by the great Jewish physician Moses Maimonides in the twelfth century, likely did little to ameliorate the disease, but almost certainly lost Maimonides some patients.
- **Ma Huang.** The active ingredient of this plant (used as an asthma treatment in ancient China) is ephedrine. It was introduced in the West in the 1920s, and while no longer a therapy for asthma, is still used in decongestants.
- **Purging and bleeding.** These radical suggestions were promoted by Hippocrates, who believed that asthma (as well as many other diseases) was caused by an imbalance in the body's "humours."
- **Tobacco.** Amazingly, soon after tobacco was brought from the New World back to Europe

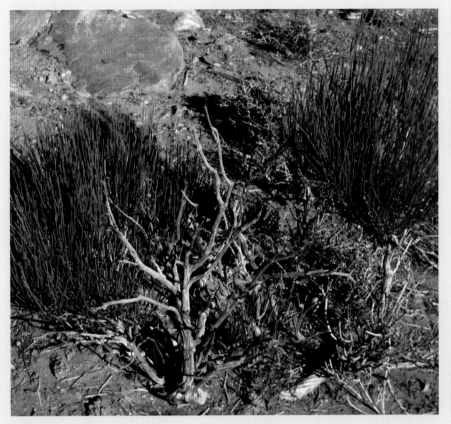

An ingredient in plants used by the Aztecs and the Chinese, ephedra was first introduced to the United States in the 1920s. Though a disappointment as an asthma medication, it continues to be used as an ingredient in decongestant medications.

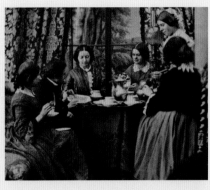

Henry Salter, a Victorian physician, recommended coffee as an asthma treatment. Caffeine is related to theophylline and aminophylline, which are effective asthma medications.

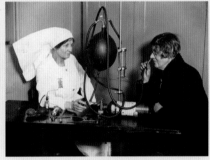

By the early 1900s, asthma-relief efforts were becoming more scientifically rigorous, as demonstrated by this early ventilator from 1919.

in the sixteenth century, smoking tobacco became popular as a treatment for asthma.

- **Stallion's dung and tincture of fox's lung.** These European remedies, extant at the same time as the above, must have made smoking tobacco seem like an appealing choice as an asthma "cure."
- **Black coffee.** Henry Salter, a Victorian-era physician, was the first to recommend this. And, in fact, caffeine is related to theophylline and aminophylline, both of which are effective asthma medications.
- **Atropine.** Extracted from the Datura or deadly nightshade plant, the poisonous atropine worked as a bronchodilator and soon gave rise to safer derivatives, such as ipratropium, that continue to be used as asthma medications today.
- **Adrenaline.** Introduced in 1900 and first used in an inhaled form in 1929, adrenaline served as the forerunner of today's inhalers, many of whose medicines (such as salbutamol) mimic some of adrenaline's actions. The modern age of asthma treatment had begun.
- **Marijuana.** In the 1920s, Grimault and Sons began to market "Indian cigarettes," containing a mix of marijuana and belladonna, as a treatment for asthma. Sixty years later, in 1980, the Institute of Medicine included asthma as one of the diseases for which medical use of Cannibis shows promise. Not surprisingly, this finding was immediately—and is presently—controversial.

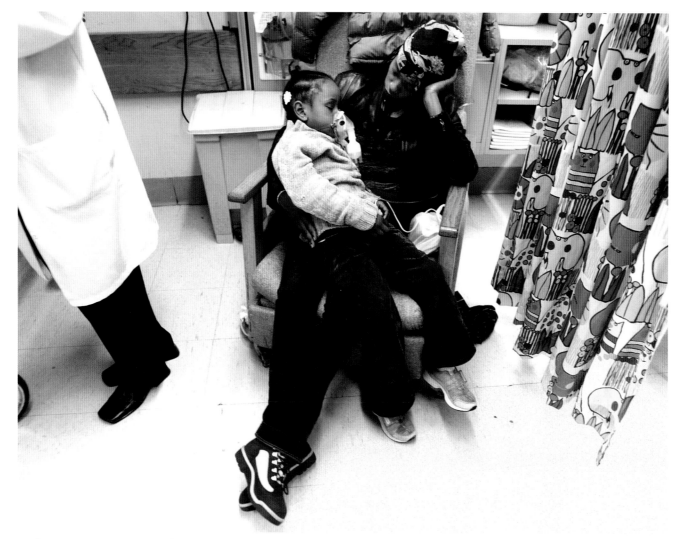

with treatment; presence of airway hyperreactivity; and, crucially, chronic airway inflammation in which a variety of different cells and cellular elements play a role. These include mast cells, eosinophils, T lymphocytes, macrophages, neutrophils, and epithelial cells.

The critical role allergies play in asthma has come to the forefront in recent years. Many allergens, including dust mites, cockroaches, pets, mold spores, and others can all spur the production of Immunoglobulin E (IgE), beginning the cascade of responses that leads to an asthma episode.

The advances in understanding the complex cellular role in airway inflammation have been matched by those of diagnosis of disease severity. The most objective indicator of asthma severity today is measurement of airflow obstruction by spirometry (FEV1) in initial diagnosis. Some studies indicate that peak expiratory flow (PEF) may also be an important tool, especially for long-term monitoring in patients with chronic asthma.

Investigators are also searching for a genetic basis for asthma. Several genes have been directly associated with asthma, including one that directs the body to overreact to allergic stimuli by creating IgE. This anti-IgE

A young asthma patient awaits treatment in an emergency room in Brooklyn, New York. For a host of reasons, inner-city children have suffered disproportionately from asthma as the incidence of the disease has risen in recent years.

monoclonal antibody is effective in patients (in conjunction with inhaled corticosteroids) with an allergic component to their asthma. At least 70 percent of asthmatics have an allergic component to their asthma; almost 90 percent of children with asthma have a positive skin test indicating the presence of IgE.

Still, much research remains to be done to pinpoint further genetic bases for the disease. In addition, while asthma clearly runs in families, studies of family history as a predictor of asthma risk have thus far demonstrated low positive predictive value.

Treatments for asthma have leaped ahead just as quickly as knowledge of the disease's pathogenesis. While beta-2-adrenergic agonists—often used in conjunction with oral corticosteroids— remain the treatment of choice for short-term management of asthma attacks, other weapons have begun to enter the physicians' armament.

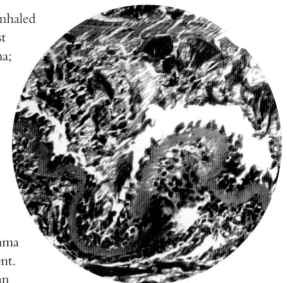

The epithelial lining of an asthmatic lung. While normally smooth, here the lining is wavy and curly as a result of constriction. Dark inflammatory cells, characteristic of asthma, are also visible.

In recent years, inhaled corticosteroids have begun to take an important place in asthma therapy. While not having the immediate effect on symptoms of the beta agonists, they are far superior at preventing future attacks. Combination therapy using the two types of treatments may provide the best maintenance results yet.

Another tack seeks to interrupt the immune cascade. Leukotrienes, compounds released by mast cells, eosinophils, and airway epithelial cells, can cause brochoconstriction, increased permeability, and enhanced airway reactivity. Recent studies reveal that these leukotrienes are involved in the pathogenesis of chronic asthma. As a result, drugs that antagonize the leukotriene pathway and have been approved by the FDA for use as maintenance therapy for mild persistent asthma, though their exact role in asthma therapy remains to be established.

In addition to pharmacologic treatments, recent attempts to reverse the rise in asthma include a combination of public education and thorough research. Preventable environmental and socioeconomic factors in asthma— such as the increased risk of allergic reactions to cockroaches in infested homes—have led to the creation of public education programs. These programs help asthma patients manage their chronic disease, which often requires several complex treatments per day. They also teach which allergens can exacerbate an asthma attack, as well as what can be done to prevent them.

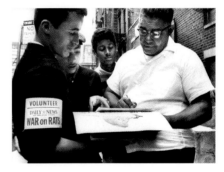

An eradication program seeks to oust vermin from homes in Harlem, New York City. Researchers have found that cockroach infestations—common in urban areas—are one important risk factor for the development of allergic asthma.

Research has also provided important insights into asthma in children. William S. Beckett, M.D., M.P.H., past chairman of the American Thoracic Society Scientific Assembly on Environmental and Occupational Health, helped design a birth cohort study at Yale University. Under the direction of Brian Leaderer, M.D., the Yale Asthma Study has followed a birth cohort for more than eight years. It has discovered that children with asthma may have more symptoms with higher outdoor air-pollution exposure, even when that exposure is below current

EPA standards. As the children in the cohort grow older, researchers hope to be able to determine how many days lost from school, doctor visits, and doses of rescue medication might be avoided if an ideal home environment can be identified and achieved.

With asthma, as with air pollution and other issues, the American Thoracic Society is using its scientific credibility and prominent membership to influence lawmakers. The Society's offices in Washington, D.C., frequently arrange for members to fly in from key districts to meet with their representatives in Washington. Also, the Society's Advocacy Network employs e-mail "Action Alerts" to urge Society members to write their senators and representatives when important bills are coming up for a vote. Successes include a letter/e-mail campaign that aided the passage of multimillion-dollar increases in Centers for Disease Control funding for pediatric asthma control in 2001 and 2002.

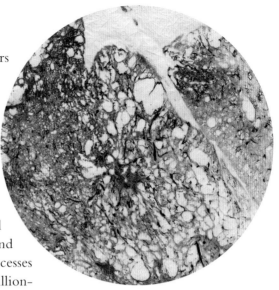

A lung stricken with emphysema. Notice that the lower left portion of the lung is darker and healthier while the right side is deteriorating.

CHRONIC OBSTRUCTIVE PULMONARY DISEASE

If publicity, legislation, and its impact on children make asthma perhaps the best-known chronic lung disease, the most obscure is easily chronic obstructive pulmonary disease (COPD). Every respiratory specialist is intimately familiar with COPD, but to the public it remains an over-looked and underdiagnosed pulmonary disease.

Depending on the definitions used, as many as twenty-four million Americans may suffer from some stage of COPD. Symptoms include cough, sputum production, shortness of breath, and exercise limitations. In 2000, nearly 120,000 Americans died from the disease, making it the fourth-leading cause of death in the United States after heart disease, cancer, and stroke. Add to this 1.5 million emergency room visits, 725,000 hospitalizations, $18 billion in direct costs, and $14 billion in indirect costs, and COPD's staggering toll becomes clear.

Emphysema and chronic bronchitis, the two major entities comprising COPD, were first described early in the nineteenth century. The French physician René Laennec dried the cut surfaces of inflated lungs in the sun to reveal lung destruction in individuals with emphysema with respiratory airspace enlargement and coalescence. These experiments helped him demonstrate the persistent overinflation of the emphysematous lung and its decreased elastic properties.

By early in the twentieth century, Orsos, a Hungarian physician, published the definitive study of ruptured elastic fibers in emphysema. His findings were followed by those of John Gough, a British physician, who described two major forms of the disease: centriacinar (which involves mainly the upper half of the lungs) and panacinar (the lower half).

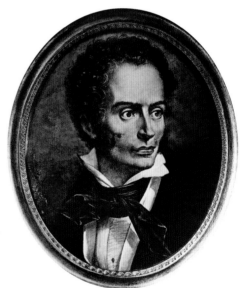

The nineteenth-century physician René Théophile Hyancinthe Laennec was the first to discover that the lungs of patients with emphysema—along with chronic bronchitis, one of the two diseases that make up chronic obstructive pulmonary disease—were persistently overinflated and lacked healthy lungs' elasticity.

Emphysema and Your Genes

ALPHA-1 ANTITRYPSIN

Most of the causes of emphysema/COPD are environmental, including smoking and use of biomass fuel. In certain cases, however, the cause is hereditary: a genetic flaw that leads to a lack of enough of a crucial protein—alpha-1 antitrypsin—in the body's bloodstream.

Alpha-1 antitrypsin, produced mainly by cells in the liver, protects the lungs by limiting the effects of a class of enzymes called elastases. Elastases are employed by the body's white blood cells. They protect the fragile tissue of the lungs by killing bacteria and counteracting the harmful effects of toxic particles inhaled into the lungs.

Elastases' protective work, though, might begin to harm lung tissue itself if not for alpha-1 antitrypsin, which blocks further action of the enzymes once the bacteria have been destroyed. In individuals with inherited alpha-1-antitrypsin deficiency, not enough of the protein exists to prevent the elastases from damaging the lungs. The result is scarring of the alveoli.

Diagnosis of inherited emphysema at first follows the same course as diagnosis of any form of COPD: medical history, physical examination, chest X-ray, CT scan, and pulmonary function tests. A pair of blood tests can then determine whether a patient's emphysema is hereditary: one test measures the concentration of alpha-1 antitrypsin in the blood, while the other identifies the actual genetic defect on the SERPINA1 gene on the patient's fourteenth chromosome.

Since 1987 an alpha-1 proteinase inhibitor has allowed patients to control the damage caused by elastases. This sterile alpha-1 antitrypsin product taken from human blood plasma and administered via intravenous infusion weekly to provide the patient with needed alpha-1 antitrypsin, has been shown in concordant observational studies to slow the rate of decline of lung function in recipients, though definitive randomized controlled trials are not yet available.

Beyond this compound, management of inherited emphysema also follows that of other forms of COPD: smoking cessation, exercise, healthy diet, avoiding

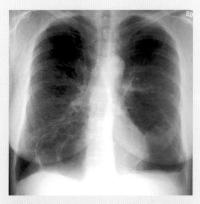

The lungs of patients with emphysema show consistent hallmarks of the disease, including dilated air spaces and loss of elasticity.

infection, oxygen therapy, and pulmonary rehabilitation. In severe cases, lung transplantation or lung-reduction surgery may be an option.

As with other genetic diseases in which the abnormal gene has been identified, investigators believe that gene-replacement therapy may one day provide a solution to alpha-1-antitrypsin deficiency. For now, that outcome remains a long-held hope, not a reality.

By the mid-twentieth century, some physicians and scientists had begun to refer to "chronic bronchitis and emphysema," instead of just "emphysema." Chronic bronchitis was defined as chronic productive cough and emphysema as enlargement of the respiratory airspaces with lung destruction. Once the two diseases were differentiated, the term COPD came into existence to describe chronic bronchitis or emphysema associated with irreversible airflow obstruction.

Today, the ATS/ERS Statement on Chronic Obstructive Pulmonary Disease continues to define COPD as a disease state characterized by airflow limitation that is not fully reversible. The airflow limitation is usually both progressive and associated with an abnormal inflammatory response of the lungs to noxious particles or gases.

It has been known since the 1950s that tobacco smoking was the major risk factor for development of COPD, with environmental and occupational air pollution and airway infection playing much smaller roles. Yet only about 15 to 20 percent of smokers develop COPD, which is best explained by an as-yet-undiscovered genetic factor.

While COPD remains unfamiliar to the public, the American Thoracic Society takes the disease very seriously indeed. Symposia at each international conference discuss the latest findings in molecular, genetic, and cellular disturbances associated with COPD; evaluate concepts in new classification and diagnostic strategies; review the social and economic impact of the disease; and examine therapeutic strategies including pharmacologic treatment, pulmonary rehabilitation, surgical approaches, and non-invasive surgical techniques.

The diagnostic standard for diagnosing COPD relies on spirometers—devices used to measure lung function. First developed in the mid-nineteenth century, spirometry had a profound effect on physicians' ability to understand and diagnose COPD in the clinic as well as the laboratory. By the mid-twentieth century, spirometry allowed researchers to use forced expiratory volume in one second (FEV_1) as a reliable measure of ventilatory function, and the ratio of FEV_1 to forced vital capacity (FVC) to measure airflow limitation.

In the 1960s, instruments were developed to measure partial pressures of O_2, CO_2, and pH in arterial blood, revolutionizing the care of COPD. The subsequent development of pulse oximeters for measuring saturation was another important advance. But perhaps the most crucial advance in knowledge about COPD has been the elucidation of the key role of hypoxemia in causing secondary erythrocytosis, pulmonary hypertension, and cor pulmonale.

Such critical findings and advances have enabled researchers to develop far more effective therapies than existed a generation ago. Unfortunately, since many individuals with COPD in its earlier stages have few or no symptoms, they don't visit their doctor to get tested. Further, well over half of all patients with COPD seek care from primary care physicians, many of whom do not use spirometers in their offices. Therefore, cases of early or moderate COPD frequently go undetected.

To address this issue, the American Thoracic Society recently joined with the American Association of Family Physicians, the American College of Physicians, and the American Academy of Pediatrics to form a Spirometry Task Force. The ongoing goal of the task force is to provide an evidence-based case that spirometry is an important tool in primary care, while also encouraging the diagnosis and correct classification of COPD and asthma through broader use of the procedure.

Further education about treatment options remains essential as well. Smoking cessation is a cornerstone of specific therapy; while smoking prevalence declined from 41 percent in 1964 to 26 percent at present in the United States, further decline will only reduce the number of future cases of COPD. For those diagnosed with the disease, stopping smoking at once is important. Those diagnosed should also receive

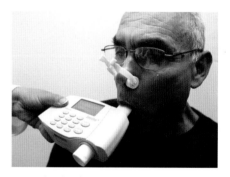

Since the development of the first spirometers—devices used to measure lung function—in the nineteenth century, spirometry has become an essential tool in the diagnosis and management of COPD.

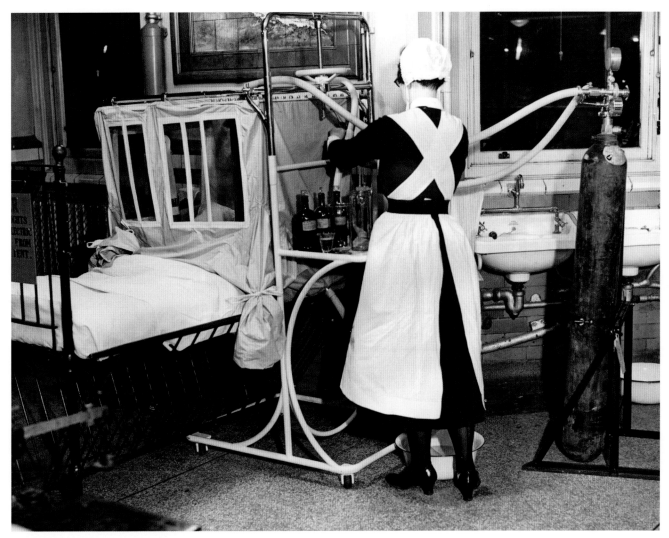

vaccinations against influenza and pneumococcal infection, while those exposed to dust or fumes in the workplace should attempt to minimize exposure by changing jobs or other means.

Bronchodilator drugs are the major element of symptomatic therapy for COPD. Use of beta-2 agonists sometimes reduces symptoms, and anticholinergic drugs also are often recommended for patients with frequent COPD symptoms. Guaifenesin, potassium iodide, and N-acetyl-cysteine are three mucolytic drugs that may provide symptomatic relief.

Among secondary therapies, long-term oxygen therapy is a non-pharmacologic option that appears to greatly benefit many COPD patients. Back in the 1920s, Alan Barach pioneered the development of oxygen tents (and continuous oxygen therapy) in treating hypoxemic patients. Decades later, the NIH's Nocturnal Oxygen Therapy Trial (NOTT) demonstrated that oxygen therapy can help patients regain significant lung function lost to COPD and other chronic respiratory conditions. In combination with rehabilitation therapy—a multidisciplinary program whose goals are to improve exercise capacity, independence,

For patients with COPD, every breath can be a struggle. Back in 1935, when this photograph was taken, long-term oxygen therapy inside oxygen tents provided an effective though unwieldy treatment option. Oxygen, now delivered through masks and tubes, continues to be an important part of COPD treatment.

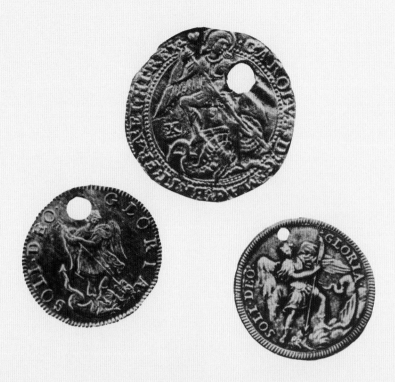

Seventeenth- or eighteenth-century coins, believed by desperate tuberculosis sufferers in France and England to contain the magic of the "King's Touch," which was believed to ward off—or even cure— the dread disease.

Drug Development: Fighting Back Against Respiratory Diseases

The search for effective treatments for disease has been one of the most fascinating chapters in the history of medicine. Until recently, the hunt seemed built on trial and error mixed with wishful thinking. "The King's Touch," for example, in which tuberculosis was cured by contact with the country's supreme ruler, must have seemed logical only to those desperate to defeat the then-incurable disease.

However, trial and error often brought success. Derivatives of quinine, used for centuries and harvested from the cinchona tree of South America, are still the first-line preventative for malaria, while the flowers of rosy periwinkle provide two alkaloids (vincristine and vinblastine) to treat childhood leukemia and Hodgkin's disease.

In still other cases, the discovery of a new drug involves pure observation and the ability to ask the right questions. In the 1910s, soil researcher Selman Waksman noticed that the soil contained far fewer disease-causing microbes than he had expected, and from this Waksman later announced the discovery of streptomycin, the first effective treatment for tuberculosis.

In recent years, however, drug discovery has entered a revolutionary new era. As scientists study the body at the cellular and genetic levels, the understanding of the causes of disease and of the body's responses to provocation have led to an extraordinary array of new treatments for respiratory diseases.

For example, anticholinergic medications have been part of the armament against asthma for centuries: Atropine, derived from the *Datura* plant, was introduced from India to Western medicine in the early nineteenth century. But in recent years scientists have learned how the chemical messenger acetylcholine causes bronchoconstriction and have developed anticholinergic medications that control airway onstruction in both asthma and COPD without the side effects of earlier atropine derivatives.

Similarly, research on cobra venom's effects on human lungs in the 1930s first identified SRS-A, a substance that appeared to mediate the development of symptoms of allergic asthma. Much later, however, researchers identified SRS-A as a set of cysteinyl leukotrienes and began to study how to inhibit leukotriene synthesis to halt the allergic process that frequently causes

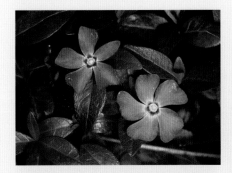

Medicines from the garden: Periwinkle has long been used in Europe to treat burns, cramps, and other conditions, while the rosy periwinkle has produced two important anticancer drugs.

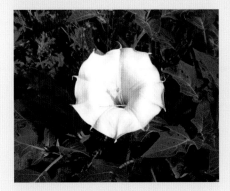

Datura, an important plant in Indian medicine for centuries, contains atropine, an anticholinergic with anti-asthma properties. Scientists continue to test plants for medicinal effects.

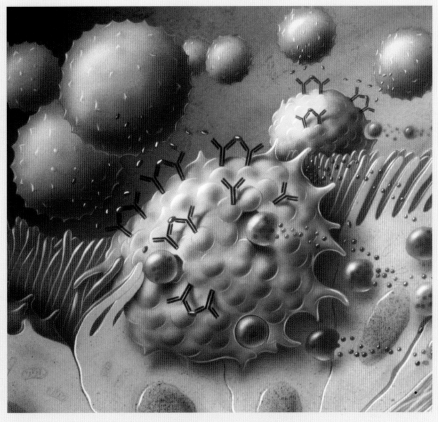

A human mast cell degranulating after exposure to grains of pollen. A deeper understanding of the complex "immune cascade" that can lead to asthma is enabling pharmaceutical companies to develop drugs that interrupt the cascade at early stages.

asthma. Today, antileukotrienes play an important role in maintenance or "controller" treatment of asthma, and have lately been shown to also speed recovery from acute attacks.

A similar understanding of cellular processes led to the development of inhibitors of other chemicals linked with asthma and COPD. Phosphodiesterase4-inhibitors, for example, block the action of cyclic nucleotide phosphodiesterases and raise the level of chemicals called cAMPs. Increased cAMP levels inhibit the inflammatory actions of a variety of cells, interrupting the process and long-term effects of COPD and asthma.

Pharmaceutical companies have also been developing monoclonal antibodies that bind to IgE, a crucial antibody in the allergic cascade. Creating monoclonal antibodies in the laboratory has led to development of anti-IgE medications, which bind to IgE on the surface of cells and prevent it from spurring allergic responses in mast cells, basophils, and others. The result is a significant decrease in allergic symptoms—and another promising weapon against allergic asthma and COPD.

In the battle against respiratory disease, trial-and-error and even superstition had their place. As the new millennium progresses, though, it is the hard science of cellular biology and the search for genetic causes of disease—coupled with spectacular laboratory advances—that will usher in safer, more effective drugs for respiratory diseases.

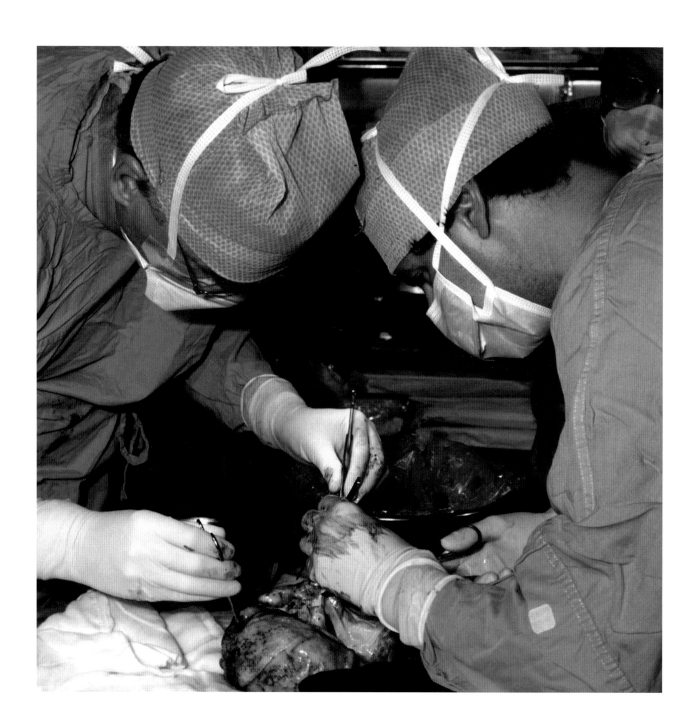

health status, and quality of life—long-term oxygen therapy is one option that can prolong life in patients with COPD.

Surgery has recently become an option for treating COPD. One procedure is lung volume reduction surgery (LVRS), first introduced by Otto Brantigan in the late 1950s. The surgery, most often utilizing video-assisted thoracic surgery (VATS), involves bilateral removal of 20–30 percent of the worst areas of an emphysematous lung by peripheral resection. Benefits include restoration of elastic recoil in the small airways, leading to a decrease in airway resistance; restoration of outward chest-wall elastic recoil; improved ventilation–perfusion matching in the remaining lung tissue; and reduced end-expiratory lung volume, which returns the diaphragm to a more favorable precontraction length to optimize pressure generation.

The most recent long-term trial on LVRS, the National Emphysema Treatment Trial (NETT), showed that the procedure yielded a survival advantage for patients with both predominantly upper-lobe emphysema and low baseline exercise capacity, while increasing the overall chance of improved exercise capacity.

In the most critical of all cases, lung transplantation may even be an option. Increasingly widely used since the advent of the anti-rejection drug cyclosporine in the early 1980s, transplants have been utilized in patients with COPD (about 40 percent of all transplants), as well as pulmonary fibrosis, sarcoidosis, smoke inhalation, and other conditions. According to the 2004 guidelines produced by the American Thoracic Society and European Respiratory Society, lung reduction surgery and lung transplantation may improve quality of life and exercise capacity in patients with COPD.

Unfortunately, oxygen therapy, pulmonary rehabilitation, surgery, and other efforts have not ended what has become a worldwide health-care crisis. While cigarette smoking remains the leading cause of COPD in the nation, the global story is starkly different, and requires dramatic changes in approach and international cooperation.

A Worldwide Partnership

In the spirit of cooperation that has transformed medicine in recent decades, the American Thoracic Society has engaged in partnerships with other, related medical societies across the United States. For example, it has worked closely with the American College of Chest Physicians on assessing asthma in the workplace, creating guidelines for cardiopulmonary exercise testing, and many other subjects. Similarly, the intertwined relationship between respiratory medicine and critical care has led to a close working relationship with the Society of Critical Care Medicine and other critical-care organizations.

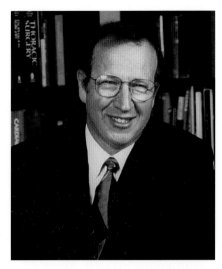

Dr. Joel Cooper, a pioneer in the development of lung-volume reduction surgery and lung transplantation, two relatively new treatment options that increase quality of life and exercise capacity in patients with COPD.

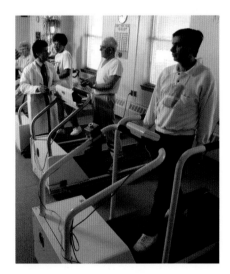

Pulmonary rehabilitation, therapy utilizing a carefully designed exercise regimen, has been shown to improve COPD patients' quality of life.

Opposite: In a procedure that could only have been dreamed of a generation ago, surgeons prepare a donor lung for transplant.

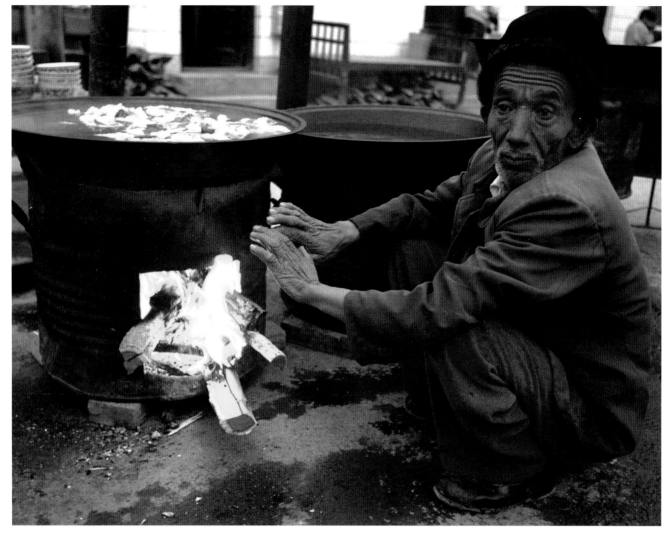

But to confront the full threat of COPD, the American Thoracic Society had to build bridges not just across the United States, but also across the world.

As it is in the United States, COPD is the fourth-leading cause of death worldwide. The World Health Organization (WHO) estimates that more than 2.75 million people die from the disease each year. In addition, though hundreds of millions of people struggle with the effects of COPD on a daily basis, it remains by far the most undertreated of the world's major killers. Public health officials estimate that as many as half of all people with the disease remain undiagnosed.

The challenge of finding, diagnosing, and treating global COPD is a daunting one, and growing steadily more so. As cigarette use declines in the United States, tobacco companies are exporting their product across the globe. Smoking rates are increasing dramatically in China and other countries, contributing to the global rise of COPD.

Other international habits will be equally difficult to rein in. Preeminent among these is the use of biomass fuel (usually wood or

While cigarette smoking remains the leading cause of COPD in the United States, a chief culprit elsewhere in the world is inhaling smoke from biomass fuel used during cooking. Here, an Uighur man warms himself while cooking mutton stew in Xinjiang, China.

animal dung) for cooking and heating in enclosed, unventilated areas. More than three billion people worldwide use biomass fuel, and as many as half a million die each year from COPD caused by it. Biomass smoke is also associated with increased prevalence of acute respiratory infections in children, lung cancer, tuberculosis, and asthma. It may account for four percent of the global burden of disease and more than 1.5 to 2 million premature deaths per year.

In response to the COPD epidemic and other global health issues, the American Thoracic Society has created the Forum of International Respiratory Societies (FIRS). The Forum's goal has been to help coordinate the efforts of a group of far-flung respiratory organizations, including the American Thoracic Society itself, the International Union Against Tuberculosis and Lung Disease, the European Respiratory Society, the American College of Chest Physicians, the Union Latinoamericana de Sociedaded de Tisologia y Enfermedades Respiratorias, the Asociación Latinoamericana del Tórax, and the Asian-Pacific Society of Respirology.

One immediate goal of FIRS is to encourage ratification of the WHO Framework Convention on Tobacco Control (FCTC) by at least forty countries. Proposed in response to the globalization of the tobacco epidemic, the FCTC would require price and tax measures, rules protecting individuals from second-hand smoke, tobacco-product disclosures, and limitations on advertising and promotion, especially those directed at children.

In addition, FIRS assists ongoing WHO efforts to improve interactions between private practitioners and national tuberculosis control programs throughout the world. Diagnoses of tuberculosis outside the United States are often made in the private sector; difficulty of follow-up may be the reason that outcomes of care don't seem as favorable as in locations where public organizations take a leadership role in tuberculosis diagnosis and treatment.

The strong international network sought by the American Thoracic Society focuses on COPD as well. This is demonstrated clearly in the organization's involvement with the Japanese Respiratory Society (JRS), which has a membership of approximately ten thousand respiratory physicians. Each year, American Thoracic Society speakers, along with members of other organizations, are invited to participate in the JRS's Congress. In 2003 the two organizations co-sponsored (with other international societies) the first meeting devoted to COPD in Asia and the Pacific Rim, which brought together health-care professionals, scientists, and policy makers to examine COPD-related problems in the region. The collaboration of the American Thoracic Society and the European Respiratory Society to create the 2004 guidelines for COPD treatment stands as another important example of cross-border partnership.

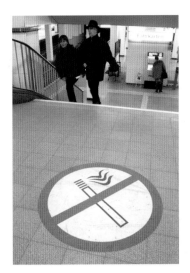

While antismoking measures have reduced smoking rates in the United States and Western Europe, efforts in Eastern Europe and many developing countries continue to lag. The American Thoracic Society is working closely with international health organizations to address that crucial issue.

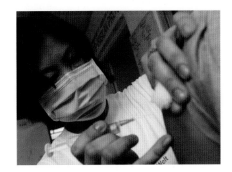

A volunteer gives an anti-tuberculosis injection in Payatas, Philippines. Haphazard administration of medication, lack of directly observed therapy, and crowded urban conditions have led to a new tuberculosis epidemic in countries across the world.

On a smaller scale, but just as important, has been the growth and development of ALAT, the Latin American Thoracic Association. When ALAT was formed in 1996 to represent the educational, research, and scientific needs of the more than 500 million people living in nineteen Latin American countries, the American Thoracic Society provided advice and logistical support. A recent ALAT president, Carlos Torres, M.D., has served as a presidential appointee to the American Thoracic Society Board of Directors.

The importance of such international societies cannot be overstated. 25 percent of the Latin American population continues to be exposed to biomass smoke. In addition, thirty-six million people in the region live at altitudes of twenty-five hundred meters or more, making research on high altitude and its effects on respiratory disease a priority.

"ALAT can offer the possibility of local research studies to adapt and validate international respiratory disease guidelines," comments Torres. "Guidelines based on local studies are better than a simple translation of international guidelines."

The American Thoracic Society's International Respiratory Epidemiology (IRE) Program, begun in 1994 and now revamped as the Methods in Epidemiologic, Clinical and Operations Research (MECOR) Program, seeks to provide the most hands-on aid possible to physicians and scientists in Latin America. It was first conceived of by then-Society president Sonia Buist in 1990, at a time when the American Thoracic Society was far less international in scope than it is today.

"The idea behind the IRE program was that there is a huge need in developing countries for health data specific to those countries," Dr. Buist comments in a piece written for the American Thoracic Society's centennial. "This need could best be met by increasing the capacity in these countries for doing studies that would inform health authorities and policy makers."

The first IRE effort was an intensive one-week course in basic and clinical investigation for twenty-five students in Mexico City. Subsequent courses have been given in Chile, Brazil, Argentina, and Peru, to students that include local physicians and public-health workers.

Over the years, more advanced courses have been added. Today, the MECOR program has four levels of courses and teaches seminars on applied clinical research methods, protocol development, data analysis, and scientific writing.

The future of respiratory medicine clearly lies with this "think globally, act locally" philosophy. The links that the American Thoracic Society have forged with international organizations will only grow stronger and more crucial in the years to come, as the battle against epidemic diseases—both familiar and new—continues.

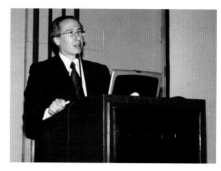

Carlos Torres, past president of ALAT and one of the many links between the American Thoracic Society and other respiratory societies. Maintaining international relationships is crucial to learning about how different conditions affect the lungs.

Opposite: Like these attendees at a village market in the Andes Mountains of Peru, thirty-six million South Americans live at altitudes greater that twenty-five hundred meters. The American Thoracic Society is collaborating with the Latin American Thoracic Association to gain new knowledge about high altitude and its role in respiratory disease.

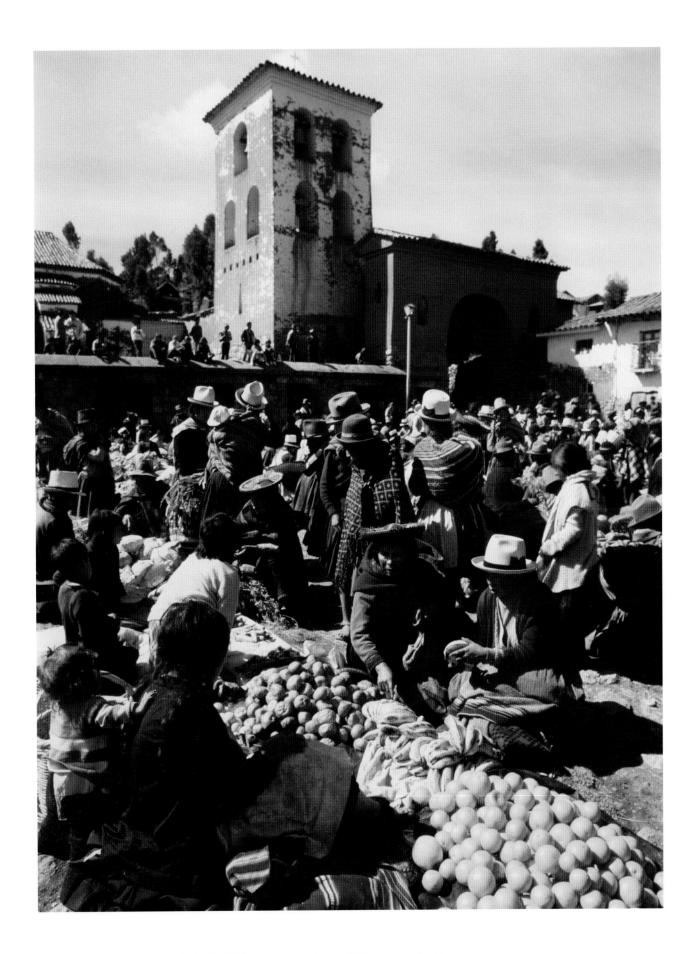

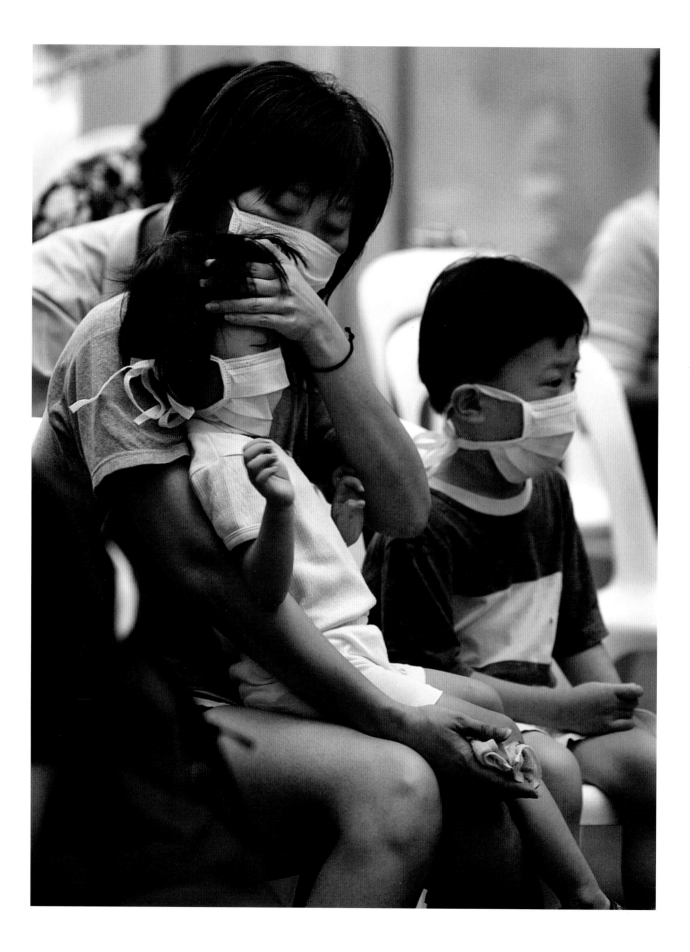

CHAPTER FIVE

Global Threats, Global Cooperation

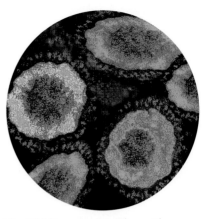

The SARS coronavirus. The rapid unmasking of the virus responsible for the epidemic disease stands as a testament to the worldwide medical cooperation needed to confront future emerging diseases.

"For in the final analysis, our most basic common link is that we all inhabit this small planet, we all breathe the same air, we all cherish our children's futures, and we are all mortal."

—JOHN F. KENNEDY, THIRTY-FIFTH U.S. PRESIDENT (1917–1963)

RESPIRATORY MEDICINE HAS NEVER been more characterized by international teamwork than it is today. In the battle against tuberculosis, COPD, asthma, HIV, other global epidemic diseases, and smoking, worldwide cooperation is the norm. Whereas the original American Sanatorium Association—the precursor to the American Thoracic Society—included only members from the United States, today more than a quarter of the Society's 13,500 members are citizens of other countries. In fact, about 40 percent of the attendees at the Society's International Conference are from outside North America and about 50 percent of the articles published in the American Thoracic Society's journals are authored by foreign scientists.

At a time when nearly every headline seems to warn of the dire effects of another hitherto unknown disease (West Nile virus, hantavirus, avian influenza, SARS), such cross-border cooperation is not only logical, it is essential. Yet, ironically, the same forces that enable scientists and physicians in New York City, the Andes of Peru, and the steppes of Asia to work closely together in the battle against respiratory disease have also provided the vehicle for emerging diseases.

One of the most dangerous of these, Severe Acute Respiratory Syndrome, or SARS, directly affected researchers and practitioners in a way not experienced since tuberculosis a century earlier. For these professionals, serving patients meant the possibility of contracting the disease, and raised the necessity of quarantine—which in turn directly affected the American Thoracic Society and its annual International Conference.

Unlike HIV and Ebola, which arose in Africa, the SARS virus made its species-to-species jump in the Guangdong province of China.

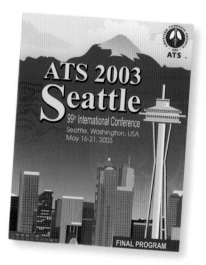

At its 2003 International Conference, the American Thoracic Society disseminated information about SARS. One important symposium, featuring leading SARS experts from China, Hong Kong, and the Centers for Disease Control, provided a vital perspective on this epidemic disease.

Opposite: A family waits in the SARS virus screening area in Singapore, one of the nations hit hardest by the SARS outbreak in 2003. By the end of the outbreak, more than eight thousand patients in thirty countries had been diagnosed, and more than eight hundred had died.

Guangdong, an intensely cultivated farming region, is a haven for emerging diseases due to its dense human population in close contact with a variety of animal species.

In early 2003 a professor of medicine traveled to Guangdong to treat an outbreak of a strange and sometimes fatal respiratory disease. The disease's course began with flulike symptoms: cough, sore throat, fever, headaches, muscle aches, and sometimes diarrhea and vomiting. In some cases, though, the illness then progressed to pneumonia, acute respiratory collapse, and death.

Here, it turned out, was exactly the kind of emerging disease that health experts most feared: one that could be spread through droplets expelled when an infected individual sneezed, coughed, or even exhaled. Worse, its incubation period could last as long as two weeks before symptoms started, during which time an infected individual could spread the disease widely.

The professor himself soon became infected. From Guangdong, he carried the disease to a hotel in Hong Kong, where he infected twelve other guests. Some of these guests spread the disease throughout Hong Kong. One, dubbed a "super-spreader," infected ninety-nine people in a single hospital, while others boarded airplanes and carried it across the world.

As quickly and easily as that, a disease that a generation ago would have flared and disappeared in a single isolated outpost—if it had emerged at all—had been given all the help it needed to become a worldwide epidemic. And for a while, it looked like SARS might become just that, as major outbreaks quickly occurred in China, Hong Kong, Singapore, Toronto, and elsewhere. But before the disease could gain epidemic momentum, stringent worldwide health efforts (centered around isolating suspected cases from uninfected individuals) halted the spread of the disease, and the SARS outbreak came to an end.

Even as the initial outbreak was drawing to a close in the spring of 2003, the possible long-term implications of an easily communicable, often fatal respiratory disease were beginning to sink in. Those planning the American Thoracic Society's ninety-ninth International Conference in Seattle, held in May of that year, were suddenly faced with the prospect of hosting a gathering of pulmonary physicians from all over the world, including areas that had seen severe SARS outbreaks.

Though some members expressed concerns about attending the conference, and a few stayed away, most understood that respiratory specialists had to be able to meet to devise the best strategies to fight the disease. Most important, members of the American Thoracic Society had to be able to meet with physicians and scientists who had personal experience with SARS.

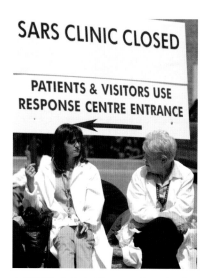

A SARS clinic in Toronto closes its doors in spring 2003, after the first outbreak of SARS had been contained. Since then, new outbreaks have occurred in China and elsewhere, and experts expect to see more in the future. Having emerged, SARS is unlikely to disappear again.

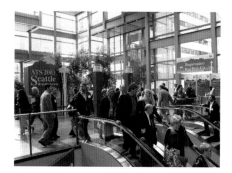

Participants attending the American Thoracic Society's 2003 International Conference. SARS, avian flu, and other emerging diseases demonstrate why the Society's global reach remains vital to the battle against respiratory diseases.

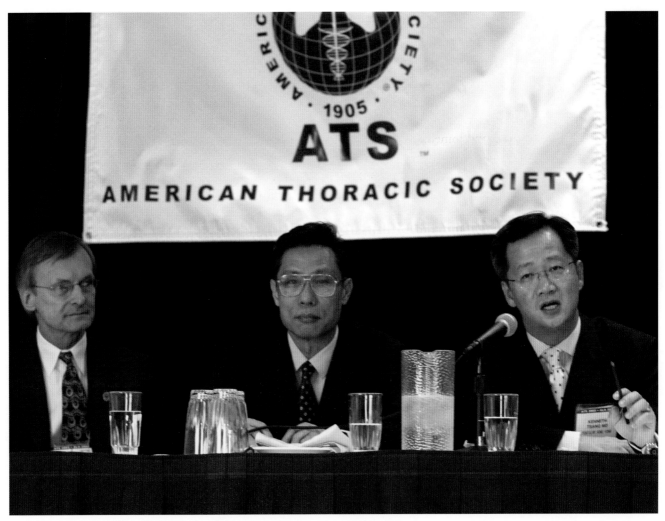

In an act that helped define the Society's role as a growing international organization, the conference featured an important symposium on SARS that brought together Nan-Shan Zhong, M.D., dean of the Medical Faculty in Guangzhou, China; Kenneth Tsang, M.D., a respiratory disease specialist at Queen Mary Hospital in Hong Kong, where the Hong Kong outbreak began; J. Todd Weber, M.D., of the Centers for Disease Control; and Jeffrey Duchin, M.D., chief of communicable disease control for Seattle and King County, Washington.

At a press conference about the symposium, the speakers were unanimous in pointing out that, though the 2003 outbreak was contained, it was impossible to know whether SARS would return. "We don't know where the disease will go next, or if there will be seasonal variations," said Weber. "Vigilance has to remain extremely high."

High vigilance will always be required for SARS—another, smaller outbreak occurred in China in April 2004, and was brought under control in June—but such vigilance is also necessary for other newly identified diseases as well. Because if one thing is certain about the future of respiratory medicine, it is that new threats are bound to appear.

Straight from the outbreak's epicenter, Dr. Kenneth Tsang (right) of Queen Mary Hospital, Hong Kong, discussed SARS at the American Thoracic Society's 2003 International Conference in Seattle. Joining Dr. Tsang were Society president Dr. Tom Martin (left), and Dr. Nan-Shan Zhong, dean of the Medical Faculty in Guangzhou, China.

Following spread: Like a dark cloud, SARS hovered over Hong Kong in the spring of 2003. These residents donned surgical masks, while others chose to take their chances without. Subsequent SARS outbreaks have been smaller and more quickly contained.

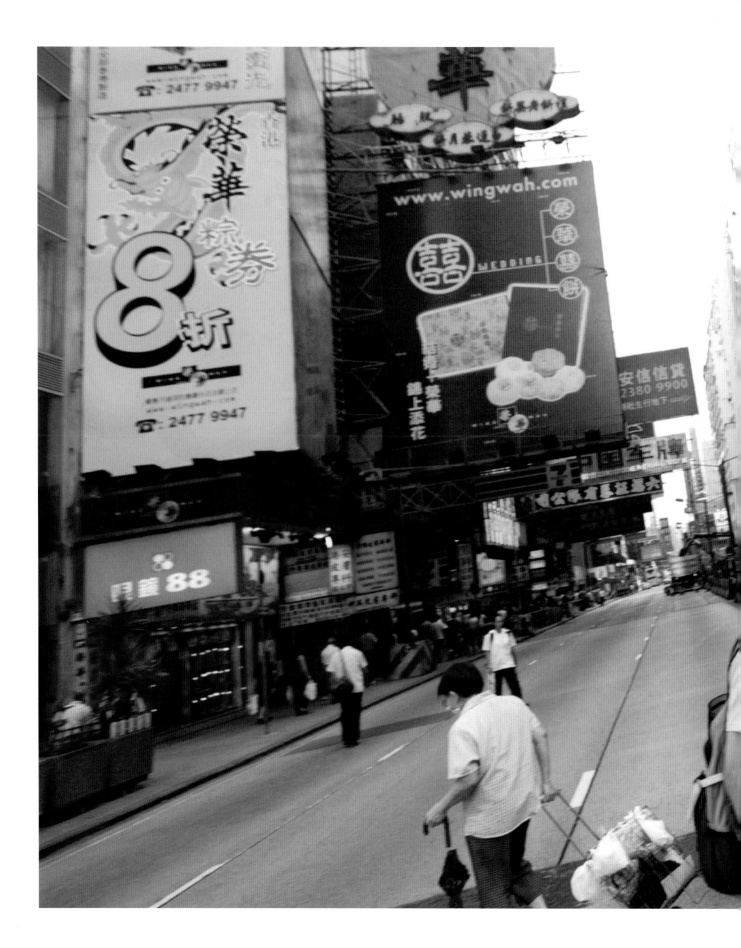

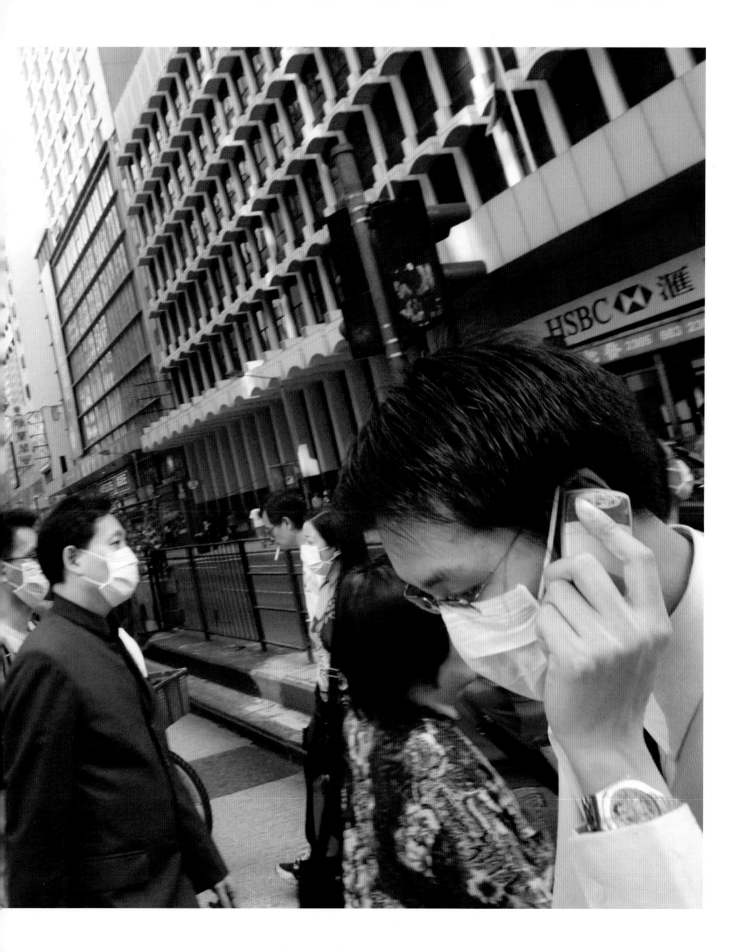

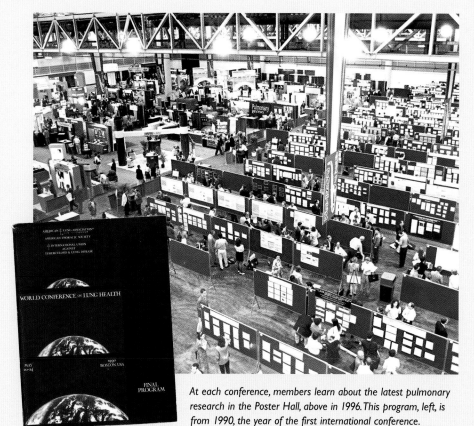

At each conference, members learn about the latest pulmonary research in the Poster Hall, above in 1996. This program, left, is from 1990, the year of the first international conference.

The American Thoracic Society's International Conferences

From tiny beginnings mighty meetings grow. When the American Sanatorium Association, later the American Thoracic Society, was founded in 1905, it had a grand total of just thirty-four charter members. These pioneers included such medical giants as Edward Livingston Trudeau, Lawrence Flick, and Vincent Bowditch, all of whom focused primarily on sanatoriums, at the time the central weapon in the battle against tuberculosis. Growth came quickly: By 1907, when the association held its third meeting,

the number of conference attendees was three hundred.

The Thoracic Society has looked outside its American borders at least since 1933, when the annual conference was held in Toronto. Since then, only two other conferences (1975 and 2000) have been held outside the U.S. (both in Canada), but the Society's efforts to expand internationally have been demonstrated in many other ways. 1990 marked the first year that the conference was officially designated as 'international.' Today, nearly 40

percent of attendees come from outside the United States and Canada, a number that reflects the global nature of respiratory diseases.

Keynote speakers at many conferences have also reflected the Society's desire to expand beyond its roots. For example, the 1986 keynote speaker was Harrison L. Rogers, M.D., president of the American Medical Association. The following year saw a keynote address by Charles A. LeMaister, M.D., president of the American Cancer Society. In 1991, the speaker was California state senator Diane E. Watson, Ph.D., the first African-American woman to serve in the state senate, who spoke on legislative efforts to reduce smoking.

The American Thoracic Society's International Conferences do more than bring together attendees from across the globe. Over the past one hundred years, the Society has provided more than 8,300 individual education sessions to physicians, scientists, nurses, and other health care professionals during its annual conferences.

Educating the world's scientific community takes vision, planning, and space: Today, with more than fourteen thousand attendees every year, the combined total of meeting rooms, lecture halls, and presentation space required to host one conference covers 10.5 football fields! As such figures show, the American Thoracic Society has become an enormous force in the battle against respiratory disease.

Express Routes Around the World: The Modern Spread of Disease

The SARS outbreak reinforced a simple fact of life today: we live in the age of emerging diseases. More precisely, we live at a time when new viral and bacterial infections are able to spread across the globe with startling— and occasionally terrifying—rapidity.

It should have come as no surprise that, as the world's population has continued to boom, other little-known or previously unidentified diseases have followed tuberculosis's lead. Additional factors, including intercontinental air travel and human settlement of previously uninhabited tropical forests, have brought humans into contact with unidentified viruses and bacteria, and have raised the risk of almost instantaneous worldwide transmission of ferociously deadly diseases.

Even in areas that have seen thousands of years of human habitation—such as intensively farmed regions of China—new diseases are emerging. Most often, these are newly evolved forms of diseases that previously affected bird and mammal species but have now jumped to humans.

The understanding that disease-causing microbes in animals might mutate to become harmful to *Homo sapiens* is not new: scientists have long believed that strains of *M. tuberculosis* may have affected fish and amphibians millions of years before the first mammal walked the earth. But again, in an age when diseases can—and do—spread from continent to continent in mere days, the concept that some previously benign, yet easily communicated, microorganism might suddenly turn deadly remains sobering indeed.

Despite tuberculosis's long history, it was a far newer disease—HIV—that brought public attention both to emerging diseases and to the ease with which they can spread worldwide. In the 1970s, the rapid increase of human settlement in the virus's sparsely populated African rainforest home enabled the virus to jump to humans. Just as important, newly built roads out of the forest to cities on each coast of Africa, ships heading to Europe, North America, and Asia, and jet airplanes with destinations across the world helped transform the disease into a global epidemic.

Today, as many as forty million people are infected with HIV globally, and thirty million have died of AIDS, a disease caused by HIV. Most cases still occur in sub-Saharan Africa, but there is no corner of the world where HIV is not present. The global village has been very accommodating to a slow-developing, fluid-borne viral disease with no cure.

AIDS is a disease that presents a multileveled challenge to respiratory specialists across the world. Complications include a panoply of bacterial *(Streptococcus, Haemophilus)*, mycobacterial (most notably *M. tuberculosis*),

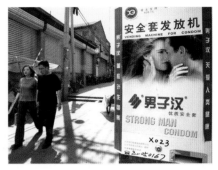

A Chinese couple walk past a condom vending machine in Beijing, part of an anti-AIDS program in China. In the 1980s, it was AIDS that demonstrated the deadliness of emerging diseases, a lesson reinforced by the appearance of ebola, SARS, avian flu, and other diseases. Preventive measures and quick containment of outbreaks remain bulwarks in confronting these diseases.

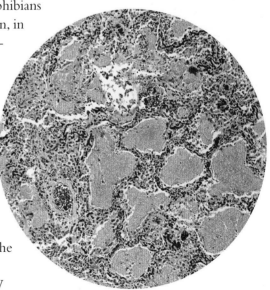

Microscopic image of a lung infected with HIV. Patients infected with HIV are prone to a host of secondary infections, including tuberculosis and other respiratory diseases.

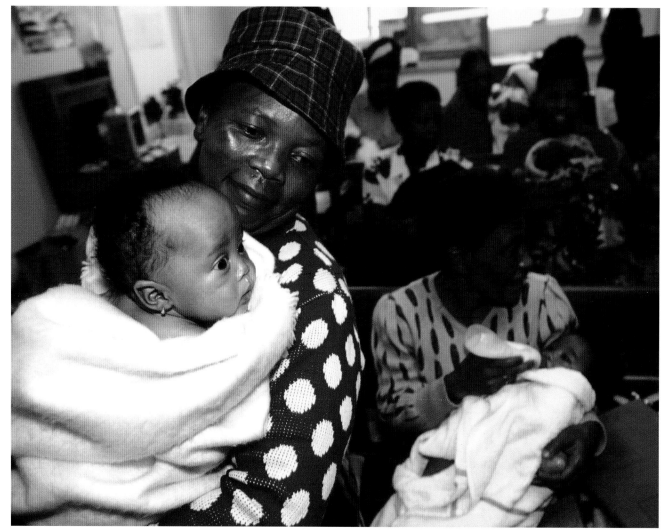

fungal (*Pneumocystis* and others), viral (Cytomegalovirus), and parasitic (Toxoplasmosis) infections centered on the respiratory system. Other pulmonary complications can include pharyngitis, lymphocytic interstitial pneumonitis, and many other infections. These respiratory complications keep the American Thoracic Society committed to finding a cure for HIV.

Despite the terrifying spread of these diseases, a modern virus has not yet developed with all the characteristics necessary for a tuberculosis-scale epidemic. Such an epidemic would require a disease that is communicated via respiratory means, can be spread for weeks before symptoms begin to show, and the human body cannot defend against.

Remarkably, one disease that currently fulfills these requirements is not a new, emerging infection. It is an ancient disease that has in recent years made a horrifying comeback across the world.

A century and a half ago this disease was considered capable of bringing civilization to its knees. Fifty years ago, it was thought to have been virtually eradicated. Today, it is once again rampaging through crowded factories, tenements, and prisons, often in a deadly new form

AIDS and its associated infections remain a global challenge, especially in Sub-Saharan Africa. This woman is just one of 4.5 million residents of South Africa who are HIV-positive or have AIDS.

that defies the most elaborate public-health efforts to defeat—or even control—it. That disease is tuberculosis.

MDR-TB: The Nemesis Takes a New Form

Just as the nineteenth century created conditions ripe for an epidemic spread by respiratory means, the late twentieth century provided an ideal opportunity for the epidemic's rebirth. And there was another, equally telling similarity: just as tuberculosis caught the attention of nineteenth-century Europe and North America only when the wealthy, the famous, and the elite were struck down, the new tuberculosis epidemic reached the public eye only when it moved from the prisons, factories, and shantytowns of the developing world to a far more prominent stage—New York City.

In the 1970s, as funding for tuberculosis diagnosis and treatment was being cut, new cases were beginning a steady rise. New York, a "melting pot" city whose poverty-stricken areas at the time differed little from those seen in the nineteenth century, was a logical hotspot. The combination of worsening poverty, the rise in homelessness, and the emergence of AIDS contributed greatly to the spread of the disease, and by 1989, when doctors had diagnosed more than four thousand cases in the city, the New York tuberculosis outbreak had reached epidemic proportions.

The epidemic was brought under control by the early 1990s, but the struggle to do so unnerved experts: the cost of fighting the 1989–92 epidemic in New York was at least one billion dollars—and that was for an outbreak that struck "only" about four thousand people a year at its height. But even this good news was tempered by something far more sobering to the physicians and other public health experts: hundreds of the New York City tuberculosis patients were suffering from forms of the disease that were resistant to isoniazid and rifampin, the two drugs most commonly used to treat it.

M. tuberculosis's ability to develop resistance to antibiotics was known almost as soon as the first effective antibiotic was developed. By the late 1940s, anti-tuberculosis regimens already included a combination of antibiotics, and by the 1990s the armament included isoniazid, streptomycin, rifampin, ethambutol, and pyrazinamide. But these New York City cases made it clear that the disease had already come close to developing strains resistant not only to baseline antibiotics, but to others as well. At once, multidrug-resistant tuberculosis (MDR-TB) ascended to the top rank of worldwide health threats.

Despite this rebirth in public awareness, the rise in cases of MDR-TB has only continued to gather momentum in the years following the New York City outbreak. People at risk of contracting MDR-TB include, logically, those who were exposed to someone with active disease, but a list

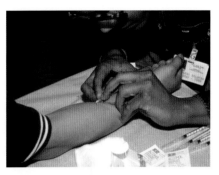

It *can* happen here. Faculty and medical students at New York Hospital-Cornell Medical Center screen New York City high school students for tuberculosis in 1992. The early 1990s' outbreak in New York City mirrored a surprising rise in cases in Europe and elsewhere.

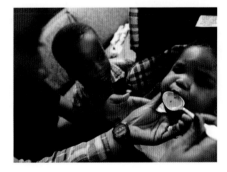

Wherever possible, use of directly observed therapy (DOT) ensures that patients will take the complex regimen of drugs necessary to cure today's strains of tuberculosis. Unfortunately, DOT remains little used in many countries where the tuberculosis epidemic continues to grow.

Not a Life Sentence

CONTROLLING TUBERCULOSIS IN RUSSIAN PRISONS

The obstacles to reversing the resurgence in tuberculosis can be seen most clearly in prisons in Russia and developing countries. These prisons, where as many as eighty prisoners may live in an airless cell no bigger than an office conference room, serve as enormous reservoirs for the ever-more-resistant MDR-TB. Not surprisingly, many of these prisoners receive lax or nonexistent diagnosis and treatment, and few patients are quarantined, leading to infection rates up to one hundred times that of the outside population.

Many factors obstruct efforts to control this epidemic. Caution against outside interference, a lack of treatment via directly observed therapy (DOT), and other issues mean that in Russia alone, as many as 20 percent of new cases of MDR-TB within its borders are resistant to all known antibiotics. Without immediate assistance, the MDR-TB problem in Russia could be a tragic repeat of the nineteenth century epidemic: a worldwide crisis without a medicinal cure.

Fortunately, help is on the way. Innovative new treatment and prevention strategies are urgently needed, and American Thoracic Society members have responded. For example, in a 1999 conference co-sponsored by the Society, James B. McAuley, M.D., M.P.H., after studying American prisons, suggested that "rapid chest radiograph screening with 'mini' 100 mm technology can be a cost-effective component of a TB control program in large urban jails." This one test can protect others from catching MDR-TB and save the government millions of dollars in treatment costs.

The Society is not the only organization to react to this epidemic: The World Health Organization (WHO) and other international organizations are working hard in Russia to confront this crisis. As the WHO points out in a statement on the epidemic: "Prisoners have the right to at least the same level of medical care as that of the general community. Catching TB is not part of a prisoner's sentence."

The WHO's Health in Prisons Project (HIPP) seeks to establish DOT as a standard of treatment for tuberculosis in prisons. Additionally, USAID has donated $34.2 million to create a program in Russia

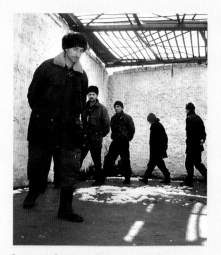

Prisons in Russia and elsewhere in Eastern Europe serve as reservoirs for the spread of tuberculosis. Crowded conditions and lack of prompt medical care encourage the spread of respiratory disease.

that treats ex-convicts and the homeless with HIV/AIDS and tuberculosis.

Much remains to be done in the renewed battle against tuberculosis. Only through the ongoing, concerted efforts of the American Thoracic Society, WHO, USAID, and other organizations will the epidemic be brought back under control, but this global response is promising.

---

of those with other risk factors is even more telling: patients who have failed to take medications as prescribed; patients who have been prescribed an incorrect treatment regimen; people suffering a tuberculosis recurrence; people with HIV and other immunocompromising conditions; and people living in areas with inadequate respiratory isolation procedures, such as prisons.

Most of these risk factors can be minimized in a city or country with a strong public health system and abundant financial resources—but not in countries where such resources do not exist. As a result, the world is now in the midst of an epidemic of MDR-TB that may be impossible to slow, much less contain.

In March 2004, a World Health Organization report gave the grim details. Eastern Europe and Central Asia have become the epidemic's hotspots, with Estonia, Kazakhstan, Latvia, parts of the Russian Federation, and Uzbekistan (along with China, Ecuador, Israel, and South Africa) reporting MDR-TB rates of up to 14 percent in new patients. This rise in tuberculosis cases in these regions goes hand in hand with an explosion in new infections of HIV. As of 2004, Eastern Europe and Central Asia have

Opposite: A child receives his tuberculosis medicine in the Philippines, one of the countries hard-hit by resurgent strains of the disease. Only through a comprehensive program utilizing global cooperation can today's tuberculosis epidemic be brought under control.

Following spread: An X-ray technician studies film on a homeless New York City resident who tested positive for tuberculosis. In the United States and elsewhere, medical efforts must focus on the homeless, the urban poor, prison populations, and others who live where epidemics frequently originate.

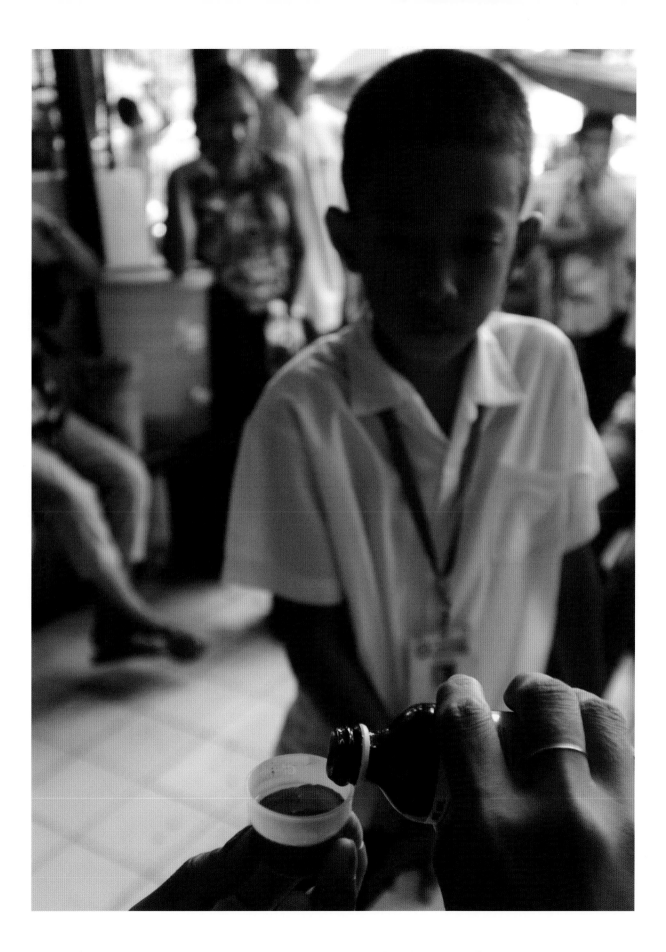

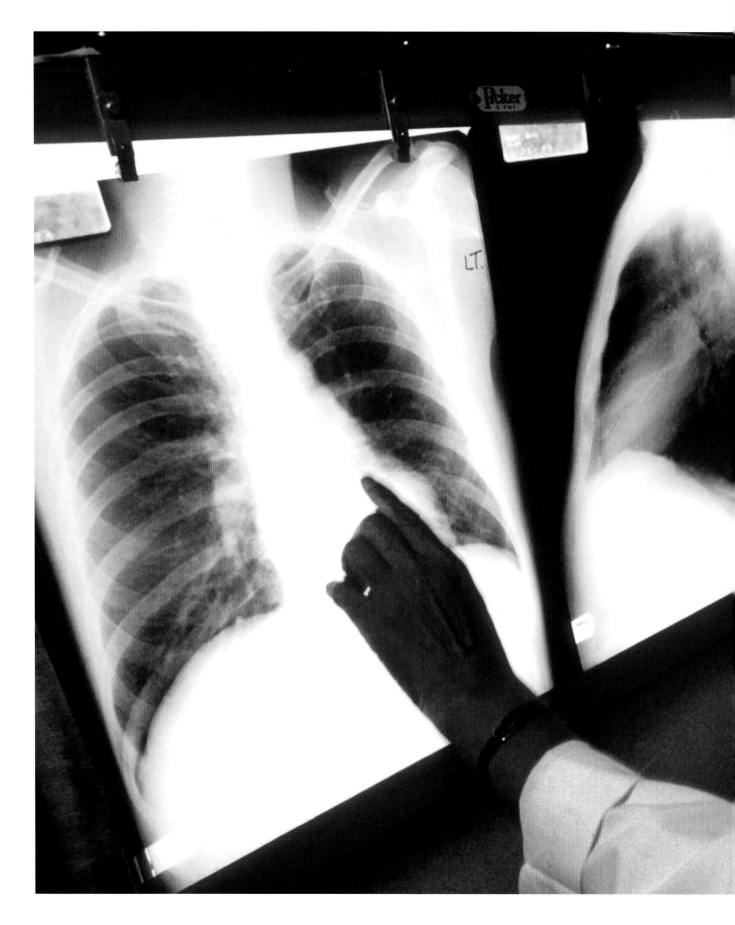

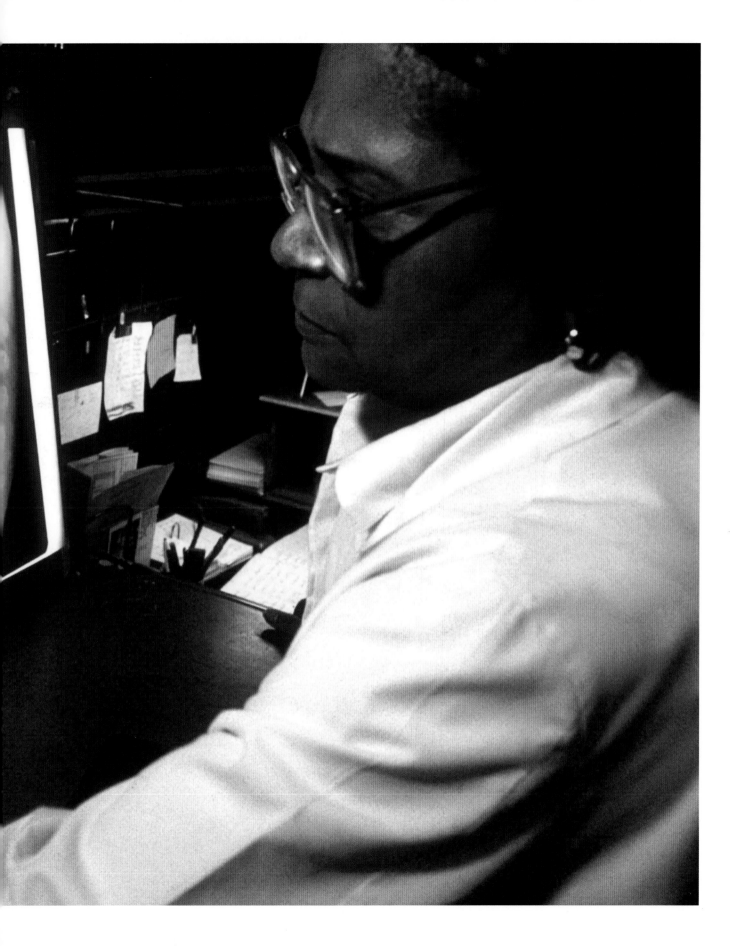

more than 1.5 million inhabitants with HIV, compared with just thirty thousand in 1995.

It is possible to gain control over the new tuberculosis epidemic. In recent years, infection rates have declined in the United States, Cuba, Hong Kong, and elsewhere due to strong, efficiently run, and well-maintained anti-tuberculosis strategies. Additionally, a single pill, Rifater, combines isoniazid, rifampin, and pyrazinamide. This makes compliance easier, while preventing patients from taking one of the antibiotics but not the others, a common route to development of MDR-TB. Further, 1998 saw the approval of the first new drug for pulmonary tuberculosis in a quarter century: Rifapentine. Designed to be taken as part of a multidrug regimen, it also offers the advantage of being administered just once a week during the final four months of treatment.

The explosive rise in MDR-TB cases and the difficulty of effective treatment make new anti-tuberculosis drugs an urgent priority. The Global Alliance for TB Drug Development, a WHO partner, is relying on both public and private research centers to build a pipeline of promising new drugs. But since public-health funding and pharmaceutical companies alike moved away from basic research into new classes of tuberculosis drugs more than thirty years ago, the road ahead figures to be a long one.

From the Gene Outward: Basic and Clinical Research

For researchers studying tuberculosis and other respiratory diseases, a deeper understanding of disease causes, pathogenesis, and treatment all depend on a return to the root of much disease process: the gene.

A generation ago, the idea of studying respiratory diseases through the human body's DNA would have seemed as outlandish as time travel. But extraordinary technological leaps in chemistry, microscopy, and imaging have allowed investigators to uncover many of the secrets of our genetic makeup.

The first, and still perhaps the most famous example of genetic research involves cystic fibrosis. In 1989 researchers first identified that a defect in the CFTR gene on chromosome 7 was linked to future development of cystic fibrosis. This discovery opened the door to an intensive, ongoing search for the genetic bases of other diseases as well.

The American Thoracic Society considers this search essential. Each international conference features dozens of abstracts, symposia, postgraduate courses, and other presentations on the basic science of gene expression; microarray analysis of diseases; and, of critical importance, the ongoing attempt to translate basic genetic findings to clinical practice.

Basic research looks to the body for answers, seeking the key to disease in cells and genes. Clinical research focuses on the patient, attempting

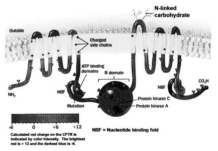

A defect in the CFTR protein, above, is now linked to the development of cystic fibrosis. This breakthrough in research is hoped to be the first of many genetic discoveries.

to cure, prevent, or manage disease on a larger level. Finding a balance between these two fields—especially when applied to genetics and cell and molecular biology—has been an ongoing topic of strong interest and debate in recent years. Claude Lenfant, M.D., director of the National Heart, Lung, and Blood Institute (NHLBI) from 1982 to 2003, was a longtime observer and participant in the subject. "During my entire tenure at the National Institutes of Health, my position has been very simple and very consistent," he says. "Basic and clinical should not be a 'pendulum.' Rather, both should be essential components of a global approach to a disease problem."

One knotty challenge to basic research is the long lag period between genetic discoveries and effective therapies based on them. Fifteen years after the cystic fibrosis gene was identified, an array of gene therapies have failed—though many more remain to be tested. "These newer disciplines need much more time to produce positive results than did physiology and pathology in the old days," comments Lenfant.

Similar challenges face researchers studying molecular and cell biology. While molecular and cell discoveries have led to more effective therapies for HIV, asthma, and other diseases, translating scientific discovery into measurable human benefit is bound to remain difficult for the foreseeable future.

At the American Thoracic Society's international conferences, participants representing all twelve assemblies address these challenges. Symposia and postgraduate courses give researchers a solid grounding in the discipline, while also exploring basic findings on molecular mechanisms of lung development, response to disease, immune response, and a wide variety of other subjects. Simultaneously, a host of presentations detail how such findings may help physicians develop new approaches to treating asthma, COPD, pulmonary arterial hypertension, and other diseases and conditions.

Another active field of research is proteomics, the study of the body's proteins. Investigators are now able to identify and analyze changes in active proteins in different cell types and under different conditions using gel electrophoresis, chromatography, and other techniques. Currently, much research focuses on applying proteomics to toxicology and drug-target identification. Ongoing studies of the proteomics of inflammation also hold great promise in treating asthma and many other diseases.

At the birth of the American Thoracic Society a century ago, debates over the proper course of medical treatment often pitted trained physicians against self-taught "medics" bearing mysterious potions and untested therapies. Today's debates are part of a larger horizon containing highly trained, determined physicians and researchers who share a common goal: deciphering the code that lies behind respiratory diseases, and using the key they find to treat and cure disease.

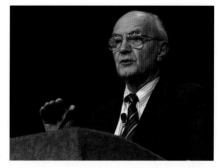

Dr. Claude Lenfant gives the President's Lecture at the American Thoracic Society's 2004 International Conference. As director of the NHBLI for more than two decades, Lenfant sought to balance basic scientific research on a molecular and genetic level with clinical research that seeks more directly to benefit the patient.

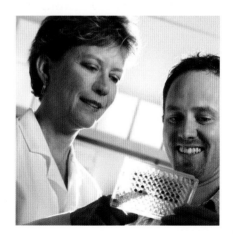

Scientists, such as Jo Rae Wright, Ph.D., from Duke University, work on solving the mysteries of lung disease, at the basic science, cellular level.

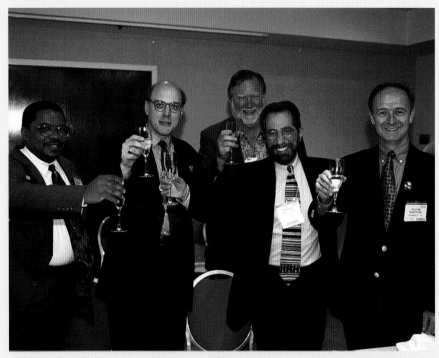

The American Thoracic Society's negotiating team celebrating the completion of the Society's separation agreement with the American Lung Association. Pictured from left to right are Drs. Talmadge E. King, Jr., Jeffrey L. Glassroth, John Stevenson, Edward Block, and William Martin.

A Break from the Past

The American Lung Association's founding in 1904 as the National Association for the Study and Prevention of Tuberculosis was quickly followed by the creation of the American Sanatorium Association, forerunner of the American Thoracic Society, in 1905. From the beginning, the two organizations were closely related, sharing much of the same membership and working together to improve treatment, education, and sanatorium conditions in the ongoing battle against tuberculosis. The close relationship was cemented in 1915, when the Sanatorium Association officially became the medical section of the National Tuberculosis Association.

In the decades that followed, through name changes and an ever-expanding mission, the American Lung Association and American Thoracic Society each played a crucial role in bringing hard science, financial resources, and public awareness to a host of respiratory diseases and their causes. The battles against tuberculosis, asthma, the dangers of cigarette smoking, COPD, and others all benefited greatly from the longtime relationship between the two organizations.

By the mid-1990s, though, sentiment was growing among the American Thoracic Society leadership to achieve some form of independence from the Lung Association. Since its founding, the Society had grown and evolved in astonishing ways: where once it had been a tiny organization of sanatorium directors, now it was a 13,500-member-strong international society with its own diverse needs and goals, not all of which were being served by its role as the medical section of the Lung Association. Clearly, change was needed—but how much change?

After ninety years together, establishing independence proved a delicate process, not free of rifts and difficult hurdles. Smaller steps—a separate mission statement for the Thoracic Society, a separate line for the Society in the Lung Association's budget—did not satisfy the desire for change. In 1997 Thoracic Society president Philip Hopewell announced for the first time in a public forum that the Thoracic Society needed to become an independent organization.

Once this ultimate goal had been announced, months of hard work remained. One critical phase took place in February 1998, during a tense, marathon mediation session in Chicago between a group of leaders of the Thoracic Society and a group from the Lung

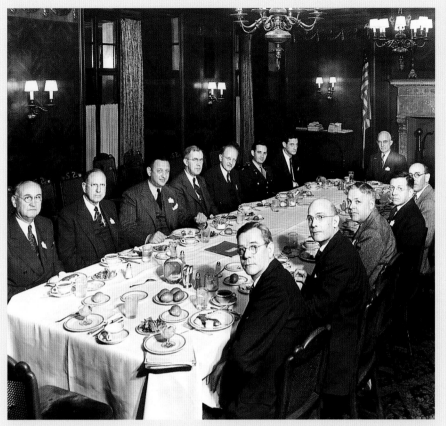

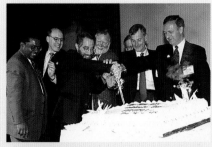

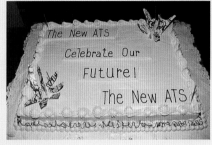

After years of discussion and months of negotiation, the split between the American Thoracic Society and American Lung Association became official in spring 1999. The event warranted a celebration of "the New ATS" in a party that June.

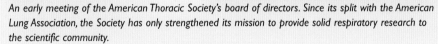

An early meeting of the American Thoracic Society's board of directors. Since its split with the American Lung Association, the Society has only strengthened its mission to provide solid respiratory research to the scientific community.

Association. Negotiators emerged from the session with eight settlement principles designed to take the first steps toward independence for the Thoracic Society.

Further negotiations over these principles occurred in late 1998 in Toronto. Here, the two negotiating teams settled on nine conceptual agreements for the separate incorporation of the Thoracic Society. These agreements soon came to be known as the "Toronto Accords."

Following further intense negotiations, final legal contracts were signed in April 1999. On January 1, 2000, the American Thoracic Society finally became what it is today: an independent, international membership organization focused on the needs of its members and their patients. "The journey to the 'New' ATS was arduous and required courage, togetherness, and determination," Edward R. Block, M.D., a member of the Chicago negotiating team and Society president during the critical 1998–99 year, wrote in a piece commemorating the Society's one-hundredth birthday. "Those of us who walked this journey will always carry with them a special sense of kinship, pride, and satisfaction about the process in which we were honored to have participated and about eventual success of our efforts."

The Future of Respiratory Medicine

The past century has witnessed a revolution in the study, care, and treatment of respiratory disease. In the early 1900s, when the American Sanatorium Association was getting its start, physicians relied on the simplest microscopes—merely being able to identify the bacterial or viral cause of a disease was considered a victory in itself. Today, scientists are using devices of almost unimaginable power to puzzle out the tiniest genetic anomalies that contribute to a host of diseases.

Similarly, a century ago, physicians were limited by the lack of effective therapies for nearly every threat to respiratory health. Rest, exercise, and diet was the best they could do against tuberculosis. Antibiotics were still forty years in the future, as were the development of sophisticated intensive care units, mechanical ventilation, and other essential tools in the battle to keep patients with acute respiratory disease alive.

Public attitudes have changed just as dramatically. For much of the 1900s, cigarette smoking continued to be a widely accepted social habit. Smokers and others ignored, dismissed, or remained ignorant of the addictive properties of nicotine and the threats of smoke, even second hand. As late as 1960, half of all American men and nearly a third of women were smokers.

Today, cultural attitudes towards smoking—not only in the United States but in many other countries—have changed so markedly as to be almost unrecognizable. No one doubts nicotine's addictive qualities or smoking's direct link to emphysema, lung cancer, chronic obstructive pulmonary disease (COPD), heart disease, and a myriad of other health threats. Offices, theaters, public transportation, even many bars and restaurants (including, as of 2004, every pub in Ireland and every bar and restaurant in New York City) are now smoke-free. A single glance at miserable smokers huddled in front of an office building in the driving rain, and it is obvious that while not completely eliminated, another heaven and earth will pass before smoking regains the cultural cachet it had half a century ago.

Yet as we marvel at how far respiratory science and medicine have come, it's equally clear that a variety of respiratory diseases remain worldwide and ever-growing threats of epidemic proportion. Some chronic respiratory diseases develop even though the incidence and mortality rates of nearly every chronic non-respiratory disease have declined in recent decades.

For example, while increasing longevity overall has led to increased total numbers of both heart and lung diseases in recent years, heart-disease rates controlled for age have been steadily decreasing in the United States. The reasons are obvious: Researchers have identified a series of controllable contributing factors to heart disease, from smoking to hypertension to cholesterol; groups like the American Lung Association and the American Heart Association have educated the general public; physicians and scientists have

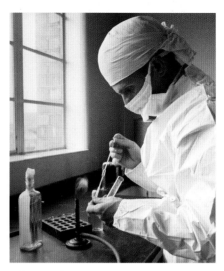

Selman Waksman's discovery of streptomycin in the 1940s seemed at last to provide a "magic bullet" against tuberculosis. More than sixty years later, however, the war against tuberculosis remains one of the American Thoracic Society's most crucial missions.

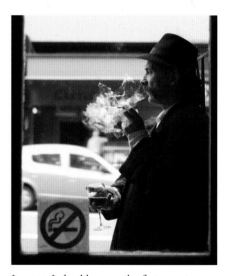

In 2004, Ireland became the first country in the world to outlaw smoking in all its pubs, restaurants, and closed public spaces. But the battle to reduce smoking rates across the globe remains one of the biggest challenges facing the American Thoracic Society.

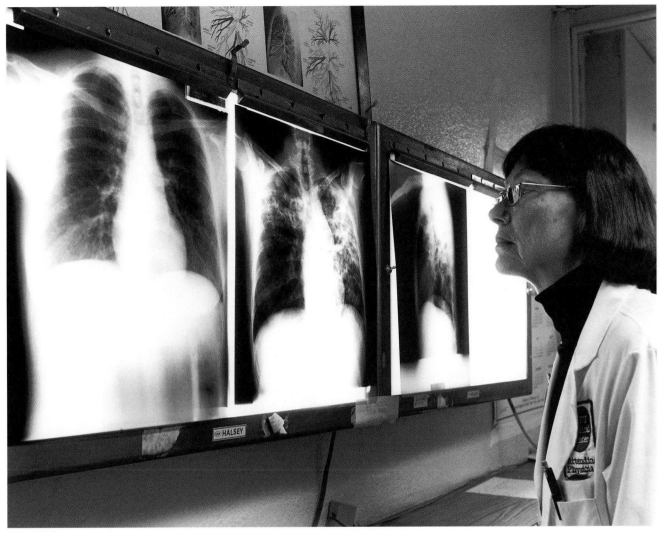

developed new arrays of drugs; and reduced smoking rates, better diets, and compliance with medical regimens have all helped reduce disease incidence.

Not so, however, with some respiratory diseases, including asthma and COPD, whose rates remain high both in the United States and worldwide. Public education and new medications have lowered mortality rates, but much work remains before the incidence of these diseases can be brought down significantly. Both asthma and COPD continue to exact an enormous toll on health, education, and the economy. Despite the American Thoracic Society's emphasis on science, more effective therapies, and methods of improving patient compliance, much work remains to be done—especially in the genetic basis of susceptibility to these diseases and the genetic basis of individual responsiveness to specific pharmaceutical agents.

Even greater challenges lie ahead on the world stage. The Society's decision in recent years to move beyond its North American borders and take on an international scope has never seemed more essential. Today, every disease is an international threat, respiratory diseases above all. This includes diseases unknown during most of the Society's first hundred years, and,

Dr. Anne Davis, the American Thoracic Society's first female president, examining chest X-rays. Every aspect of scientific technology, from the simple X-ray to the most advanced scanners, surgical techniques, and ventilators, will be employed to battle respiratory diseases old and new, from tuberculosis to COPD.

without doubt, diseases that do not yet even exist, at least among humans. Coming hard and fast during the past decades, hantavirus, Marburg, Ebola, West Nile, SARS, and other viruses have proven once again that the battle against respiratory disease is an ever-evolving struggle. Protecting the public from these emerging diseases will require quick identification as well as massive public-health and education efforts.

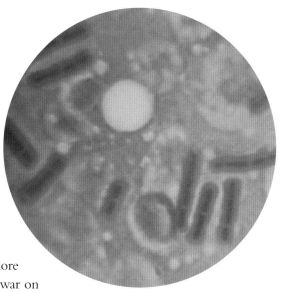

The anthrax bacillus, magnified one thousand times, is a rod-shaped cell with square ends. When anthrax-laced letters began to appear in 2001, bioterrorism became the newest front in the war against respiratory diseases.

Opposite: Doctors in New York train to respond to bioterrorism. Today's doctors are prepared to face a number of new challenges.

But new diseases are not all that have emerged during the past few years. The attacks of September 11, 2001, soon followed by letters laced with anthrax in Washington and elsewhere, have made respiratory specialists especially important in the modern age.

As the September 11 attacks proved, terrorism can have a respiratory component. But the anthrax letters demonstrated even more strongly that respiratory medicine has moved to the forefront in the war on another threat unheard of during much of the Society's first hundred years: bioterrorism.

Bioterrorism, once merely a frightening possibility, is now a reality. Soon after the anthrax attack, the American Thoracic Society created a task force chaired by Mark Frampton, M.D. The goal of the task force was to mar-shal the Society's resources *before* another attack: to determine who among American Thoracic Society members had expertise in the pulmonary effects of bioterrorism, and who might be interested in joining the effort.

What began as the Society's bioterrorism task force has become a full-fledged Section of the Assembly on Environmental and Occupational Health. Perhaps most crucially, the Section did what the American Thoracic Society as a whole has been doing in recent years: it reached beyond its borders. Meetings among the Society's members, scientists from the National Institute of Allergy and Infectious Diseases, and officials from government agencies represented a crucial new step in the war against this new "disease." Cross-disciplinary colle-giality has never been more important than in the post–9/11 world.

A century ago, the nascent American Sanatorium Association stepped to the front lines in the struggle to learn about, treat, and cure tuberculosis. It proved itself willing to shuck off old prejudices, ignore outdated methods, and look to the future instead of the past.

Today, as it enters its second century, the American Thoracic Society and respiratory medicine as a discipline are again center stage. In an age when many of the most serious global health threats are respiratory, members of the Society must step to the front lines once more. Both within the United States and abroad, they must serve as a rapid-response team, combining basic science, translational research, public health, education, and patient care into an aggres-sive, effective, cohesive whole.

If the past hundred years are any indication, these are challenges the American Thoracic Society is well prepared to face.

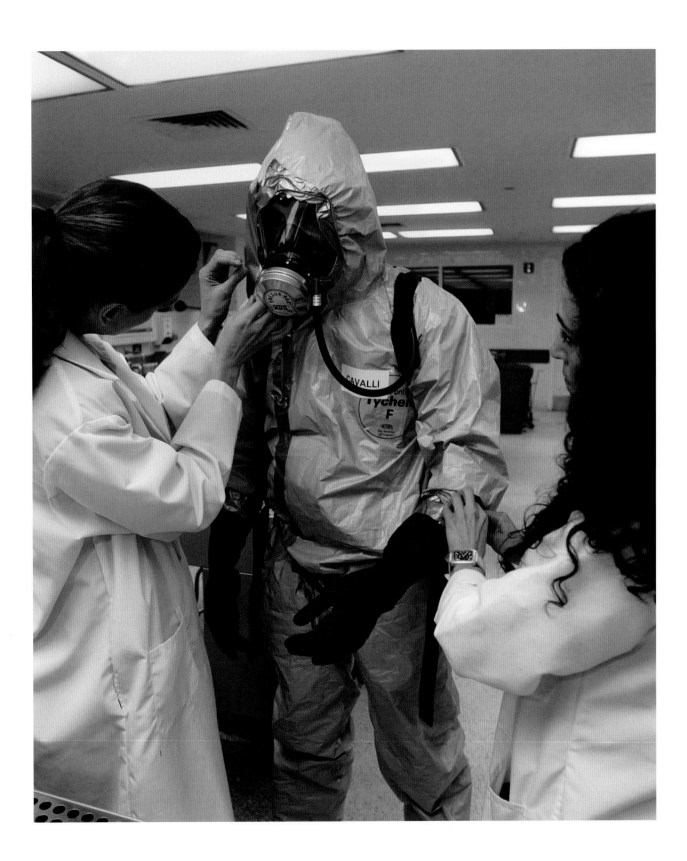

ABOUT THE AMERICAN THORACIC SOCIETY

thor-'ra-sik *adj. (ca 1656)*: **relating to, located within, or involving the cavity between the neck and abdomen in which the heart and lungs lie.**

One hundred years ago, a group of physicians and scientists formalized the collegial partnerships they had developed around the treatment of one epidemic disease: tuberculosis. They knew that in order to offer their patients the best hope for comfort, improvement, and possibly even a cure, they must share their knowledge with other medical professionals. This was the beginning of the American Thoracic Society's fight against lung disease.

Established in 1905, the American Thoracic Society has grown, flourished, and—most important—adapted to the advancements and new challenges in medicine over the last century. Today, as the American Thoracic Society celebrates its one-hundredth birthday, it is an international professional and scientific society focusing on all areas of respiratory and critical care medicine with a membership of 13,500 from around the globe. These members help prevent and fight respiratory disease through research, education, patient care, and advocacy, and are committed to the Society's long-range goal: to decrease morbidity and mortality from respiratory disorders and life-threatening acute illnesses.

Today, the American Thoracic is proud to be:

- a leading force in the fight against disease and illness

- a champion and protector of the highest scientific and research ideals

- an advisor and partner to the world's leading disease-fighting organizations

- a catalyst for ensuring that science's research is translated into practical, effective, clinical practice

- a creator and disseminator of globally recognized clinical practice guidelines

- an advocate and voice for health care professionals and the patients they serve

- an influence for change in the state of disease globally and the state of health care nationally

The most visible recurring activity of the Society is the planning and production of its International Conference. This yearly conference has become the premier forum for all physicians and scientists who work in pulmonary and critical care medicine. The attendance at this meeting has steadily grown to reach over fourteen thousand attendees each year with almost 40 percent of attendees from outside North America.

The American Thoracic Society has also created three highly respected journals: the *American Journal of Respiratory and Critical Care Medicine®* *(AJRCCM)*, the *American Journal of Respiratory Cell and Molecular Biology®* *(AJRCMB)*, and its newest journal, the *Proceedings of the American Thoracic Society®* *(PATS)*. The Science Citation Index ranks the *AJRCCM* and the *AJRCMB* first and second, respectively, among respiratory journals. The journals further reflect the diversity of the Society's membership, as one-third to one-half of published articles are submitted by non-U.S. authors.

As the American Thoracic Society begins its second century, it continues to fight against lung disease and promote lung health. While physicians and medical scientists around the world are challenged by the resurgence of diseases such as pneumonia, multidrug-resistant tuberculosis, and SARS, the American Thoracic Society continues to set the standards for prevention, treatment, and control of these and other serious, life-threatening diseases.

For more information about the American Thoracic Society, contact the Society's Communications and Marketing Department at 212-315-6442.

INDEX

PHOTO CREDITS

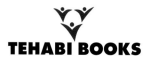

TEHABI BOOKS

Tehabi Books developed, designed, and produced *Colleagues in Discovery: One Hundred Years of Improving Respiratory Health—An American Thoracic Society Perspective* and has conceived and produced many award-winning books that are recognized for their strong literary and visual content. Tehabi works with national and international publishers, corporations, institutions, and nonprofit groups to identify, develop, and implement comprehensive publishing programs. Tehabi Books is located in San Diego, California. www.tehabi.com

President and Publisher: Chris Capen
Senior Vice President: Sam Lewis
Vice President and Creative Director: Karla Olson
Director, Corporate Publishing: Chris Brimble

Senior Art Director: Josie Delker
Designer: Kendra Triftshauser

Editor: Katie Franco
Editor: Sarah Morgans

Proofreader: Dawn Mayeda
Indexer: Ken DellaPenta
Consultant: Barron Lerner

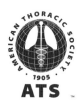

ATS

American Thoracic Society Staff

Executive Director: Carl Booberg
Director of Communications and Marketing: Cathy Carlomagno
Chief Corporate Relations Officer: Graham Nelan